Sh*t Happens

or

Around the World in 80 Dumps a Day

J E Turley is a young teacher and writer who poos into a permanent stoma bag. He wrote and narrated Sh*t Happens to raise awareness of Crohn's and ulcerative colitis, to stay sane while doctors chopped his insides out, and because his mum told him to.

His short story *You Sh*t in a Bag* was shortlisted for the International Perito Prize and published in their 2020 Anthology. Freelancing, he has words in The Focus News, Fen & Field, among others.

He loves hash browns.

Praise for Sh*t Happens

'Dark sense of humour and positivity… Keep talking about this, awareness is so important – you're helping more people than you know.'

Molly Grace – NHS

'Somehow both laugh-out-loud and thought provoking in equal measure.'

Lottie Palmer

'I love the wry humour and brave spirit of these chapters! Absolutely brilliant and an essential publication.'

Tracey Warr – Author of the *Conquest* trilogy

'Hilarious. Captivating read.'

Kathy Emms

'Well, my curiosity is finally satisfied… I'll say it again – J E Turley is an amazing writer.'

Chandrayan Gupta – Author of the *Radha Bose* series

'Fab, funny and honest read. Wish it was longer!'

Stephanie Redlick

'Amazingly brave with a wicked sense of humour. I cried and laughed in equal measure.'

Eileen Butterworth

'I started reading this, meaning to read it bit by bit, but could not put it down! It is very funny, very sad and the description of being in hospital is very realistic! Write some more!'

Sandra Collins

'King of words. Beautifully written and made me chuckle.'

Tom Golledge – Author of *Last of the Balinskis*

'Fabulous writing. Made me smile throughout and the self-deprecating humour was a hit.'

Lester Rivett

'It's a shame the chapters have come to an end... Really glad your hard chapter ended in a positive way. Look forward to reading some more of your adventures.'

Stuart Dovey

'Very rewarding to share your journey... I could identify with my own.'

Deb Beck

'So refreshing to read such an honest account of what life has dished out... these topics never get talked about and we all feel that we have to portray a perfect life – which no one has.'

Val Kemp

Sh*t Happens

or

Around the World in 80 Dumps a Day

First Published 2021 by Track Press Books
Track Press Books, 4 Penny Court, Worley Road, St Albans, AL3 5NU

Copyright © J E Turley 2021

The right of J E Turley to be identified as the author of this work has been asserted by him in accordance with the Copyright, Designs and Patents Act 1988.

All rights reserved. No part of this publication may be reproduced, stored in a retrieval system, or transmitted, in any form, or by any means (electronic, mechanical, photocopying, recording or otherwise) without the prior written permission of the author.

A catalogue record for this book is available from the British Library.
ISBN: 978-1-7399430-0-4

This book is sold subject to the condition that it shall not, by way of trade or otherwise, be lent, hired out, or otherwise circulated without the author's prior consent in any form of binding or cover other than that in which it is published and without a similar condition, including this condition being imposed on the subsequent purchaser.

Printed and bound in Great Britain by Mixam UK.

To respect the privacy of those who might not wish to be recognised, I have altered various personal details and anonymised names.

Although, sod knows why – some of you reading this are well aware of their real identities.

Contents

Welcome to it   11

Series One
1. '*O Pato*'   14
2. A Very Local Prison   23
3. 'Cover your Balls'   29
4. Mr Toilet   39
5. Wu Wang the Poo Man   44
6. '*Ah, merde!*'   51
7. Bionic Bum Fun   56

Series (Number) Two
1. Same Sh*t, Different Surgery   70
2. Lost the Plop   75
3. Loo-ful Meditation   81
4. The Final Flush   86

Open Letter:
Mental Health & Misinformation   100

Acknowledgements   109

Welcome to it

I'm fond of exaggerating. Prone to it, in fact. Bloody obsessed with it! Ok, maybe not. Enough of that. But I am acutely aware of my tendency towards the extremes of a story and the importance that you, the reader, can trust me as a storyteller.

So, I'll come clean now. The title of this book has fallen foul of hyperbole. Shit does happen. One hundred percent true. And I *have* been around the world. Not all of it and not the whole way, but enough that we can say that that part's mostly true, too. So, what's left? Eighty dumps a day? Eighty?! Ridiculous, surely? Well, I promised I'd come clean, so I'll admit my guilt in over-egging that last part of the title. You probably sniffed it out anyway. But it's got a good ring to it. And we'll soon see that it's not quite as far from the truth as you might imagine.

This is a story of shits and giggles and cries and shits. Of steroids and soul-searching, of lovers and loos. Twenty-three may seem too young to be offering up a memoir, but as I await major surgery, I know my life can't and won't roll on again until I'm close to twenty-four. What I can do is stop and take stock. And do my best to entertain you with stories of what's happened so far.

SH*T HAPPENS

At the time of writing,* next week I will undergo an operation known as a colectomy. This removes the entirety of my large bowel, or colon, leaving me with a bag for life (technically an ostomy) instead of a functioning bottom. A bit like Kim Jong Un, apparently.† The difference being that I, however, don't incite much fear with my violent and tyrannous nature outside the lavatorial domain. A toilet pot despot, at worst.

There is no known cure for ulcerative colitis. However, body minus colon equals no colitis.‡ Since every course of medicine has failed me (or vice-versa, depending on how you wish to view it), I'm up for the chop.

To trace the origins of the painful, pooey path to this sticky situation, you'll need to let me reverse your clocks to 2013. To a world where no one knew Donald Trump as anything other than a keen golfer with a name fitting to this story.§ Once there, allow me to transport you to Rio de Janeiro, Brazil, for a story of near-death natural wonders, lesbian love affairs and, most significantly, ducks...

---

* July 2019

† Kim Jong Un is rumoured, in his demi-god status, to be untarnished by base human functions such as defecating.

‡ The suffix '-itis' indicates inflammatory disease, so colitis means 'inflamed colon'.

§ YouTube 'Ali G and Donald Trump'.

Series One

Chapter One: 'O Pato'

Seven hours until I have my bionic bum fitted and there's little hope of sleep. Nightingale Ward in St Thomas' hospital should rather be called Nightinhell. Or, more simply, just Nightmare. Groans of pain from nearby beds are masked only by the incessant whirring of breathing apparatus attached to the old boy directly opposite me. In another bay out of sight, someone's drip feed has run out and will beep, beep, beep, beep until the night nurse has time to attend to it.

I don't want to be(ep) here. I want a functioning digestive system and to be somewhere exotic like New Zealand or Newcastle, Blackpool or Bermuda. And I want to be outside. (Beep.) Up a mountain or wake-boarding the sea front or hacking through the jungle. Instead, I'm up shit creek. Lost my paddle about a year ago. But it's not worth moaning. I always wanted to win Wimbledon and I've got over that not happening (yet). I'll get over this unhappy relationship with my colon soon enough too, I'm sure. Then I'll go to those places and do those things. But I promised you a story about somewhere I *had* been, so let's trace back to the lavatorial launchpad

'O PATO'

and start the countdown... 3, 2, 1, thunderpants are go!*

Rio de Janeiro, Brazil, 2013

Red flags hung a foolish stickman struggling in the *perigo correnteza*. Warned of these dangerous currents, he was swimming and getting nowhere, encircled by his sign. Winds intermittently fluttered fabric and bent the flagpole but stickman was stuck and you could see why he was being paraded as an example for all at Copacabana beach. Fearsome, towering waves rose and lashed out at the shore, full of hunger for an ignorant *gringo*.† Now, I'm no seafaring surfer, breaker of waves (...first of his name), but I'm no fool either. Today was not a day for improving my swimming.

It's called sand because you find it where the sea meets the land. Rio de Janeiro was the land of Christ the Redeemer, who had blessed us with extraordinarily cheap tickets to ride the cable car up to his lofty abode this morning. What he hadn't mentioned on the invite was that the clouds enclosing him until lunchtime made it impossible, at 10am, to see far past his knees, let alone his head. And

---

* The Gaelic name Turley means 'like Thor', or more fittingly, 'like Thunder'. YouTube 'Thunderpants trailer'.

† Gringo = European, favela = slum, bunda = bottom.

SH*T HAPPENS

you could forget about sweeping panoramic views of Rio; the exotic metropolis encased within forests flush with life; *favelas* with a frightful glamour to them, violence and corruption set to the Sugarloaf backdrop of beauty; and of course, the Atlantic Ocean, dotted with outrageously enormous peachy beachy *bundas* glistening golden in the sun, visible even from the mountains… possibly. I'll never know. Because I couldn't see a bloody thing.

Sunday service complete ('thou shalt not be a stingy bastard'), on the return leg of the cable car I was singled out as a young *gringo* and dragged to the front of the carriage to dance with a busking Samba crew. This involved standing awkwardly and smiling as seconds slow-danced into minutes, me noticeably rhythmically challenged[*] and a head taller than the performers, before putting 10 *Reais* into their donation bucket for the privilege of the forced entertainment, praying to cloudy-nuts that they'd leave me alone after that.

Down through the city, through blocks that could have been Paris, could have been London, could have been New York and out across a front street that couldn't have been Blackpool but could have been Barcelona and, at last, we had arrived at Copacabana beach. Three weeks in the outback of the country with my girlfriend's family, under the disapproving

---

[*] These days, Brazilian dancing ranks among my favourite party tricks.

eye of her Evangelical father. A morning under the mockingly invisible and chuckling belly of Christ, but now I had, finally, been redeemed.

Land ended at the sea and today so, too, did any possibility of further exploration. The waves created a double defence against aquatic entry. Huge giants crashed down – rippling smaller, secondary waves to lap a preliminary warning at the shore. Franciele wasn't a big fan of open water in any case, but with some gentle persuasion we were soon semi-submerged at a safe waist height. Me, wearing my new shades on which Fran had splashed out a whopping £14 in River Island pre-trip and her, stunning in a bikini bought on the same spree, paddling slightly shallower but more submerged. Christ, she looked gorgeous. She was a good foot shorter than me but that didn't stop me stooping for a kiss.

But I didn't make it. As long as my toes curled in the sand I'd felt we were safe. You remember that bollocks about the sea meeting the land. One of the great towering giants was decidedly dissatisfied with two teenage upstarts ignoring his foot soldiers and waded into battle. And then, my feet no longer touched the sand. Which way was up was up in the air and under the water and an indiscriminate limb flailed against something and then my head resurfaced and we were no longer paddling.

I'd lost my glasses. Fran hadn't lost her bikini, before you go getting any ideas. But we'd both lost control in an instant. Neither of us could touch the bottom and we were now fighting with every ounce of panicked anaerobic energy to return to the shore. Kicking and flailing towards safety, I was on a treadmill ramped far beyond my top speed. The wave inexorably dragged backwards, briefly dropping us down before flinging head and limbs up and hard down under the surface. Kicking up, I was the weaker swimmer but Fran didn't seem to be having any more luck fighting the giant. We both repeated this rag-doll cycle two, maybe three more times, me screaming, 'Heeeelp!' and her, '*Ajuuuuda!*' through salty breaths but both knowing our voices were hopelessly drowned beneath the giant's flurry of aquatic fury.

The closest I had to a plan B was to swim to Fran and hope that our combined mass was somehow more likely to be flung to shore. Desperately flimsy science, but plan A was only serving to sap our energy. Rising for the fourth or fifth (or sixth?) time, instead of fighting the backwards pull I went across and with it. Reaching Fran just as the giant tugged downwards, this had the inadvertent appearance of me grabbing and pulling her under the surface. Her eyes bulged with fear and confusion. Demented and bulging as mine must have also been, maybe she thought I was trying to kill her. There was no time to explain. We were under. Holding on. Spinning. Holding. Kicking. Kicking each other. Hitting something. Upwards. Kicking. Clueless as to whether in the right direction. The safe direction. The shallow

'O PATO'

direction. And then, sand. Digging my heels in, as the secondary wave feebly tried to exhort me back to the depths, I was safe.

But somewhere in the kicking and flailing and spinning we'd been separated. Where was Fran? Not near me. I turned and coughed 'Help!', spluttered '*Ajuda!*'... Two lifeguards were comparing bronzed biceps and didn't hear me, oblivious to the tragedy unfolding before them. Her looking at me like I was trying to kill her could be the last look from Fran's beautiful brown eyes, alive. What if, inadvertently, plan B *had* killed her? Saved me, and killed her. No, no no no no no no. I stepped back towards the giant as he crashed down his next thunderous blow and realised with an almighty sigh of relief that he had only been hungry for a foolish *gringo*. Now I was out of grasp, he coughed up Fran, disinterestedly, and receded. We dragged each other to the sand that was safely land and decidedly *not* sea, both falling to all fours. Coughing sea water and snot, I tried to apologise but Fran was gone. Storming up the beach, leaving her *gringo* fool collapsed centre-stage before the towering waves. The lifeguards clocked her as she passed and watched just below waist height for a moment, before returning to their biceps.

.....

Brazilian buffets are the stuff of a hungry teenager's dreams. Chicken, sausages, steaks, flavoured rice, flavoured dust (odd but *uma delícia*), beef or chicken lasagne (as a side!), potatoes, salad

SH*T HAPPENS

(I'm told), and desserts ready as soon as your savoury palate is sufficiently satisfied. I was permanently hungry. Five minutes after breakfast I was already craving lunch and today lunch arrived after a trip to the murky heavens, a tumble roll of the dice with death, and five *hours* in waiting.

So, the buffet was welcomed with both open arms and gullet and I chewed my way to an excellent value for Fran's father's *Reais*. I popped upstairs to the loo after finishing my fourth savoury plate and again after my sole dessert bowl. I never have been much of a sweet tooth. As I pootled back down the stairs for the second time, Evangelical father cracked a joke which brought a chuckle across the table at my expense. My Portuguese was in its infancy at this stage, so I asked Fran what was so funny as I plopped back into my chair, wondering if it was too weird to go back for a bit more lasagne (the beef one) post-dessert and poo.

'They've given you an *apelido*, a nickname – *O Pato* – The Duck.' Apparently I'd disappeared to the loo within minutes of eating every meal for the last three weeks. Apparently ducks do that, too. So, I was the *Pato*. I really never thought much of it before then, but I suppose I *did* always need to rush off after a meal. But it hardly affected my life. I didn't pay it any thought. And it didn't seem to bother Fran.

Later on, darting through Rio's night markets to the seclusion of the beach, we snuck a moment away from her father's not-quite-omniscient eye to finally share the kiss the sea had earlier stolen from us.

'O PATO'

But this *Pato* nickname was perhaps the first sign of my dumping deviance. Maybe, if plan B had saved only Fran and not me, the repercussions of my untimely death could have saved hundreds of miles of loo roll, Atlantic oceans-worth of toilet flushes and thousands of pounds of NHS funds. But it didn't. And I'm living to tell the tale in Nightmare Ward, the story almost dreamy in its now distant nature.

But wait, you say. You promised near death and ducks, and you delivered. What about our lesbian love affair?

Well, as may have come across in the tale, I was wholly smitten with Franciele. I moved away to university a year before her, missed her terribly and all my new friends could tell. My college football team even adapted a version of 'In the jungle, the mighty jungle… ah-wim-boh-wey, ah-wim-boh-wey' to sing 'She's his girlfriend, Bra-zilian girlfriend…' in homage to my besottedness.

And then, one year on, she followed me north to a nearby establishment and promptly forgot I existed by the end of her freshers' week. Classic! Except, contrary to the standard break-up, one year on we were best friends once more. She hadn't left me for an upgrade, rather a different product altogether. Just as we were curling our toes in the sands of her new life and our new friendship, I was both sad and happy to be a part of it. But it wasn't to last. Storm-New-Girlfriend thundered into her town, giant waves of jealousy swept Fran out to sea and this time, she didn't return to me.

I, however, did return for my final year at university to a new chant of 'She *was* his girlfriend, Bra-zilian girlfriend…'

And, while writing this, I've crept two hours closer to the mighty surgery. I should try to sleep.

Chapter Two: A Very Local Prison

I was a happy, if fiercely competitive, child. As long as I was winning, I was content. Which obviously wasn't all the time, but the pursuit of victory kept me occupied, whether in tennis, monopoly, or even just year seven French vocab tests.

That competitive streak subsided (to some extent) so sanity could remain for adulthood. With maturity, which teaches very quickly you can't always win, can't be the best at everything (or anything, in most cases) and also that you can't have everyone like you.

You have to pick your battles, or at least work out what they are. I was happily plodding through these uncertain steps into my twenties when disease struck and suddenly life was no longer about figuring out a sense of purpose. It was about survival.

Happy-go-lucky character that I've always been,[*] the idea of self-harm, that someone could or would ever choose to slit their wrists open, had always been incomprehensible. That was when life was plain sailing, before this year. Now, just as the waves had almost got me and Franciele in Rio, I was drowning

---

[*] For fans of Only Fools, YouTube 'Del Boy talks about Grandad'.

again. Each time the disease receded for days or weeks, I rose to a rasping breath of false hope that I was going to reach the shore. Then that inexorable pull wrenched my gut upside down and inside out and crashed me, flaring, back into submission.

Someone who *was* very close to me said this disease had changed me. Harsh, hurtful, but true. Before the struggles of these toileting twelve months I'd never had suicidal thoughts, never understood or even experienced depression at all.

I lost a quarter of my body mass. Lost the ability to sleep for a year. Lost the freedom to be confident anywhere more than a few metres from a toilet. Lost my energy and my patience. My body was no longer a marvellous machine, the highly functioning product of aeons of Darwinian refinements. It was a prison. Run-down, with bloody, dodgy plumbing.

Asides from the insomnia, steroids give me the shakes. Lying alone in the dark, dank, mould-peeling bedroom of my old flat after another early-hours race to the bathroom, I observed my wrist quivering in the semi-light of another morning of this new normal – this semi-life. And I understood. When you are held hostage to your health, be it mental or physical, trapped in your body, it makes perfect, terrible sense. Those blue veins tempt. There, at the surface. They offer a way out.

Thankfully these thoughts were rare. That same person who claimed the disease had changed me more frequently accused me of being all too painfully

A VERY LOCAL PRISON

positive about my condition than so morbid. I had only experienced this – this very local prison – once before. It was a snapshot of pain to come...

Durham, UK, 2014

My eyes are open, but my body refuses to move. Invisible forces hold me down as if in a vice, stock-still. Nothing supernatural, don't worry. I'm a physics student, after all. But something is seriously wrong inside. Every ounce of energy has been consumed by this illness the last few days. Now, I must be exhausted. Spent fuel rods. Alive, but incapable of movement. No, I must move. Because I will need to reach the loo again at some point all too soon.

I try to calm my panicked breathing as that is only wasting precious joules. My tennis bag and some loose clothes provide cushioning as I half-roll, half-fall to the floor. Pivoting takes two minutes or two hours, I couldn't tell you. The crawl to the toilet is similarly intemporal. Something tells me water will help stimulate some vigour within. Still on all fours I reach up and grapple for the shower knob. Turning it, I fall with two hands in the basin and the spray splatters forgivingly on my hunched shoulders, dissipating the paralysis. I can move. I can stand. I can sit back on the loo. Wash my hands then more water on my face. Then back to bed.

Fortunately, I only woke up in this state of terror that one time. But that bout of the standard fresher flu possibly wasn't so run-of-the-mill. Seven weeks into a new life at Durham, recently made friends don't know you well enough to notice the difference between a hangover and an extended period of deterioration. But I returned home for the Christmas break having lost over a stone, despite already being slim. Unknowingly, I had experienced my first flare of ulcerative colitis.

I didn't see a nurse, didn't see a doctor, barely saw a human at all for those dark, drained hours in my college room. Telling myself it was fresher flu and that I didn't need to get help. The only form of care I received came from the lovely local ladies who cleaned the college rooms. A small minority of public-school pillocks (Durham attracts a few) treated these women with as little attention and care as they did their rooms and their parents' bank accounts, but I was truly grateful for their presence in what sometimes seemed quite a lonely new life at university.

.....

In a parallel, more recent scenario, under the NHS' care this last year I have met more incredible nurses, doctors and support staff than I could possibly ever thank individually. The jobsworths really are a rarity. Unfortunately, one of the first days out of surgery my nurse really failed to act. Could she not tell from hours of agonal cries that, my epidural having failed, paracetamol wasn't quite taking the edge off open surgery recovery? I was a prisoner first

A VERY LOCAL PRISON

to the disease, then to pain, and currently to weakness and incapacity. But the shore is now, at last, in sight.

Of all the NHS workers, without a doubt my favourite (and the only person who inspired me to enter a 'Staff Star of the Month' nomination) was once again a cleaner, named Dorota.[*] Loud and always laughing, in her European drawl she would either call me 'Darling' or spoke 'Jaack' as if there was an extra vowel sound. I could have had more trips to the toilet in a night than minutes asleep and I'd still look forward to Dorota popping by for a little chinwag while she changed my bed. If I follow this kind lady's endless excitable and enthusing advice, then my first fifteen holidays after recovering will all be to places I can't pronounce in Poland. And I'll be drinking lots of bison grass vodka with apple juice. One morning she was very confused to find me on speakerphone to the police[†] and in the end just joined the conversation, with the now equally bemused officer, as I compiled a victim statement.

Sorry if this has been a darker chapter than the others so far, but these last couple of weeks have been rougher than I ever could have envisaged. The surgery is done now and, after two weeks in Nightinhell, I left hospital this evening. The next tale finds me naked

---

[*] This name actually hasn't been changed.

[†] My bike was stolen the day before I was admitted to hospital. Sh*t happens.

SH*T HAPPENS
and aggressively whipped in a sauna by a curious (and equally naked) Latvian man, so stay tuned for some lighter entertainment…

Chapter Three: 'Cover your Balls'

My first car cost £200. A navy-blue Ford Fiesta that may have been older than me. The suspension only worked on one side, causing a tilt which carried the passenger closer to the road surface. It got me to Bristol and back, to school and back a few times, and to Blackpool and back before an MOT sentenced it to die.

After less than three weeks together, the party was over and the old Fiesta was consigned to the scrap heap for £100. Amongst my mates at Nicky B Academy, the fact I had a car – any car – was a privilege, because we all knew getting a motor wasn't the pricey part: having parents who would fork out two grand for a teenager's insurance was the real barrier. So, I was lucky, and the Fiesta was my Ferrari.

Riga, Latvia, 2016

'Audi saloons are kinda poor. Like a desperate teenage boy whose family don't really have any money.'

What? Was this girl nuts? If I'd shown up at sixth-form in an Audi A4, people would have thought my dad had won the lottery. But then, my lift from Riga airport should have warned me of this.

SH*T HAPPENS

I don't have many opinions about cars; if I'm honest, they bore me. However, ever since I was run over by a four by four in St Albans a few years ago, I've decided there should be some form of extra test to prevent useless yummy-mummy- or twatty-daddy-drivers from getting behind the wheel of an off-roader. My new girlfriend had bought me flights to go and visit her, so should I really have been surprised when she collected me from the airport in an enormous Range Rover? Maybe not. But she'd only passed her test *the week* I arrived.

As we drove out of Riga to Jelena's parents' house in the suburbs, she explained that her father had chosen this particular location to build their dream property as it was the only direction in which you could leave the city without passing any Russians. As far as I could tell, 'Russian' is synonymous with 'poor' in the Latvian thesaurus. This was a route out of town that didn't pass any pre-fab tower blocks thrown up in the Soviet era. No Russians, few Audi A4s and certainly, certainly, no Ford Fiestas.

I started to wonder where I'd come and, frankly, who I was dating. This overt materialism and snobbery is viewed in England as ugly, as classless; Durham rich kids' purposefully dirty, worn-out Reeboks say it all. But I was too swept away in the novelty of Jelena, her family and of Latvia to worry too much. I soon realised that, to my hosts, I, too, was a great novelty.

'COVER YOUR BALLS'

In an accent I can only recall as something of a cross between Borat and Vladimir Putin, Jelena's father, Ernests,[*] quizzed me on everything from Oasis and the royal family to London taxis and why 'sheeps' don't huddle in British fields. Her mother asked me about tea. And her little brother asked me about all sorts, in crisper English than most seven-year-olds back home.

I was carted in the Range Rover from historical site to fancy restaurant to area of natural beauty. I'd been told to bring my best clothes for a treat her father had planned. Back at the house, I donned my (ironed!) shirt, smart shoes and black chinos and was ready for the evening's surprise entertainment.

Their house was palatial. Beautifully designed, spotlessly clean. They even had a cook. Latvian food is delicious, and I made sure nothing the chef prepared ever went to waste. The problem with that was, of course, that 'O Pato' came out to quack and I was constantly in fear that the acoustics of a spacious property (with no subtly placed loos) meant certain echoes rippled through the house. My pristine image as the English gent they were all so eager to impress was in danger.

Toilet-trouble aside, I'd inadvertently had a wardrobe malfunction too. Coming downstairs,

---

[*] Again, Jelena and Ernests aren't their real names, but if anyone can get in touch explaining why I chose these Latvian names, I'll be impressed.

ready to leave, unintelligible Latvian words were exchanged between father and daughter and I was quickly whisked up to his dressing room and given a blazer worth a good few multiples of my first car. *Jā*, now I was presentable for the opera. Yes, the opera...

The Latvian opera house is an undoubtedly impressive building; the champagne and nibbles during the interval were tasty; and above all, the seats were comfortable enough for a good kip during the show. Jelena tried to claim she appreciated it, but in a rare moment when my eyes fought the droop, I caught *her* napping! So, even posh people don't really like opera. Ha!

Naturally, I thanked her parents for the night and gave the blazer back gratefully. The next day, Jelena informed me her father had prepared another traditional Latvian experience for us – the sauna. The basement of their beautiful home was a boutique spa of sorts: sun loungers and drinks tables; the corner of the open area housed a wooden slatted log-fire sauna with a glass door.

That sounded great, but I hadn't brought my trunks and I'd feel too awkward borrowing those from her dad.

'*Nē*, silly, you don't wear anything in a Latvian sauna.'

But hadn't her mum been using the sauna earlier? I couldn't go naked in front of her mum!

'*Nē, mamma* already used the sauna today. Don't worry.'

'COVER YOUR BALLS'

So, Jelena and I descended the steps to the basement, dropped our towels on a lounger, and hit the sauna. I'd never been in one before, and was pleasantly surprised. Ten minutes in the heat, rub a rough honey-like mixture over our skin, then chill on the loungers drinking sap from local trees. A few cycles of this and I was feeling loose as a moose. All good for your health and skin too, apparently. What's not to like? Bliss...

Polishing off another glass of the slightly sour, but not unpleasant, tree sap, I was admiring Jelena – bare and beautiful – laying atop her towel on the adjacent lounger when, to my horror, the door to the cellar opened. A pair of green Crocs appeared and, worse, began descending the steps. The Crocs were attached to two hairy legs, and there was nothing at all covering the rest of what those legs were attached to. Jelena's naked father muttered something to her and disappeared behind the steamed-glass door of the sauna before I'd had time to scramble beneath my towel.

'What is he doing here?? I thought you said we'd be alone!'

SH*T HAPPENS

'Did I? I said my mom[*] had already used it today. He's just here to do the traditional Latvian sauna experience for us.'

What? I'd thought the honey scrub and weird tree drink had been the traditional sauna treatment. What was her dad here for? Could she not see that I was naked? That *she* was naked, too?

'So I'm going to be naked in front of your dad? That's normal is it?'

They must be having me on here.

'Honestly, Jack, he'll think it's strange if you make a big deal out of it. It's just Latvian saunas – everyone's naked. You'll be lying on the bench anyway. Don't be weird about it.'

With that, she reclined in her lounger and closed her eyes. Conversation over, clearly.

Five unnerved minutes later her father emerged, sweating, and asked, 'Who is first?' Jelena ushered me in without sitting up and I cautiously crossed the spa, taking my towel to protect my modesty for the walk.

Once inside, Ernests beckoned for me to lay across the longest bench, possibly amused by my reluctance to drop my towel. While he fiddled with some birch branches in the corner of the sauna, I laid out my

---

[*] Jelena's English was an American English. This may help you if, like me, you enjoy trying the accents when reading the dialogue.

'COVER YOUR BALLS'

towel and swiftly planted myself face-down across the slats. He could see my rear. A bum's just a bum, after all.

So, here I was. Naked, face-down, craning my neck to work out what was in store for this 'traditional' experience. It looked like my girlfriend's dad was dipping some tree branches and leaves into the steaming water by the door, but his backside was blocking my view so I wasn't entirely sure.

How on earth had I ended up here? I missed England and I missed Fran's nice, normal, non-naked step-dad. I wanted to laugh at the absurdity of the situation but there was no one to laugh with.

'I drip water from leaves on you and you tell me when feels same temperature as your skin. Otherwise can hurt.'

Excuse me, what can hurt? I tried to focus on the temperature but my senses were at sixes and sevens. Clueless, I obliged.

'Yeah.. I think that's the same temp-'

I hadn't finished my uncertain sentence before the very certain blows began. Ernests was a man possessed, thrashing me repeatedly from the soles of my feet, up my legs and back, all the way to my neck, jolting my face into the wooden slats of the bench. Up and down, up and down, the whipping blows of the tree branches rained on me for an indiscernible number of seconds or minutes, who knows? And, blimey! The pain. I was gritting my teeth to keep from crying out. Maybe I hadn't judged the water temperature right or maybe this was his twisted, twiggy way of saying, 'This what you get for ******* with my daughter.'

Either way, when the thrashing stopped I was just thankful the whole bizarre experience was over...

'Sit up.'

...Or was it? Now was the moment of truth. Ernests was dipping his branches and leaves in the steaming water, preparing for round two. Jelena had said he'd find it weird if I tried to hide anything or acted awkwardly. So, sitting up, I left my safety blanket, my towel, and faced him.

My girlfriend's father turned back towards me, watered weapon in hand. Everything I'd encountered in Latvia had been nuts. Now I faced a pair at eye-level.

'Cover your balls with one hand.'

I did as instructed.

'Raise your hand.'

I assumed he meant the other hand, unless this was some humiliating joke. Actually, either way this must, surely, be some kind of humiliating joke.

One armed raised, the thrashing recommenced, now from my waist, up and down the side of my torso, up and down the underside of my arm.

'Switch hands.'

The same on the other side. Sweat was dripping off Ernests' flapping naked body from his exertions in such heat. And then, finally, thankfully, he stopped.

'COVER YOUR BALLS'

'Now go outside. Temperature difference is good for the... holes?'

'Pores.'

'*Jā*, good for the pores of your skin. Stand outside maybe five, ten minutes.'

It was over. What are you supposed to say? What was the courtesy here?

'Okay.

...Thank you.'

I took my towel and left the sauna. Jelena didn't notice me or stir from her semi-slumber on the lounger. Riga during Easter is by no means commando-kilt weather and after two or three minutes I was, quite literally, freezing my nuts off. In my twenty years to this point, I'd never paid any attention to the health of the pores of my skin. After my first experience of doing so, I decided it wasn't worth the hassle. Blue-balled, I returned inside before the later stages of hypothermia set in.

Re-entering the basement, Jelena was gone. I looked to the sauna but the glass door was opaque with steam. Was she in there? What about the naked-bush-ninja? I didn't have to wonder for long. Sitting back on the lounger, I could soon hear the swoosh of my girlfriend's dad brandishing his branches. I could hear the whipping of the leaves on her naked body. And, worse, Jelena's temperature gauge was clearly as faulty as mine. The pain. With each slap on skin,

SH*T HAPPENS

there followed a high-pitched, almost carnal, yelp. Crash. 'Aaargh!' Thrash. 'Aaargh!' Whip. 'Aaargh!'

This was traditional.* This was normal.

This, however, was not for me.

There was me, worrying about what my girlfriend's family, so wealthy and well-presented, would think of my tyrannous toilet escapades in their echoing acoustics. I really shouldn't have worried. By the end of our traditional Latvian sauna experience, I knew Ernests far more intimately than I'd ever expected. I also knew Jelena's father-daughter relationship was rather more intimate than I ever plan to have with my future children.

Nevertheless, I'll conclude this story with an English phrase I'd taught Jelena walking through the market square in Durham a few weeks earlier: 'Each to their own.'

---

* Many friends have questioned if this is, in fact, a traditional Latvian sauna experience or whether I was being played. For evidence, YouTube 'Latvian sauna happy new year 2014'.

Chapter Four: Mr Toilet

Weaning off the steroids once again, I'm reminded daily of the meaning of the term 'invisible disability'.

In the aftermath of surgery, seconds bled into minutes and minutes scabbed over before they ever became hours or days. The flow of time congealed and clotted. All I wanted was to be here, now, back where I am at home today. To have dreamt of this I'd have needed to sleep. But pain is a vice of consciousness, and sleep was as intangible as health or home.

Whereas waves of agony and nausea acted as relativistic stoppers to time – constantly feeling ultra-alert and conscious of each moment's pain – stopping the steroids has the opposite effect presently. Time flies and I am caught – lethargic and inert – as it passes before me. In hospital I bristled with anticipation for all the things I would do once I was free of the disease. Now I'm out, I don't have the energy to fulfil any of these ambitions!

But it's not all bad news. The previous three times I reduced my steroid dose, the disease returned with a furious flush of vengeance. Now my large intestine is somewhere in the bins out the back of St Thomas' hospital, colitis no longer has any leverage to start another battle in World War Loo.

As one of the great (footballing) minds of our day has plastered across his neck: *'Tudo passa'*, Portuguese for 'Everything passes'. Neymar may be better known for silky skills and strange, saucy tattoos of his (admittedly) pretty sexy sister, but his neck artwork is a source of ink-redible inspiration for me. Soon, the side effects of the countless dirty drugs my body has tussled with these last thirteen months will fade. And then, I'll return to my job as a secondary school teacher, a trade I learnt in the north-east of England…

Gateshead & Middlesbrough, 2017

I sprint the length of the corridor as my tie flaps and slaps my face. Pupils are given a bollocking if they don't walk sensibly, or if they don't wear their blazers, but thankfully they're all in classrooms, as are their senior teachers, some of whom still don't realise I'm a colleague, not a sixth-form student.

My suit jacket is back in my classroom, along with my (fittingly) bottom-set year seven group and my mentor, Adam, who said he'd watch over them whilst I dash. Where to? *Quelle surprise. Les toilettes!*

Whoever designed the school clearly thought it'd be amusing to multi-task, attempting to break the world record for longest corridor while they were at it. The passage from the science department to the nearest loo was so bloody long they'd managed to

MR TOILET

install a poster along the wall tracking the entire history of humankind and the universe.

Fortunately, this school had some archaic creationist religious tendencies. So, the poster ended when god made the universe and all things bright and beautiful a mere few thousand years ago. This meant the poster (and corridor) were approximately 0.00004 percent of their true length.

But I wasn't complaining. I may not agree with the decorator's loose relationship with science. My loose bowel movements, on the other hand, most certainly did. At last, I had reached the toilet.

.....

Crohn's and colitis are invisible diseases. So invisible that I didn't pay attention to the signs until the disease had spiralled beyond hope of recovery without surgery. When I look back on 2017, fatigue was the silent symptom. Disappearing to sleep in my car between lessons, I rushed to the loo so often people would just assume I was there again. I forced myself to be busy and constantly on the move, as normal, but if I ever paused and sat down for five minutes it was a losing battle between my eyelids and gravity. So much so, in fact, that the plonker prancing around the education lecture hall every Friday made it an unfunny running joke that I couldn't stay awake during his talks. (Good one, mate. Shame your lectures weren't as riveting and original as your banter.)

SH*T HAPPENS

The plethora of ex-teachers on TV plying their trade as comedians means you will probably have heard some terrible stories about what we get up to while the kids sit exams. For example, the pac-man style game where you chase the other examiners around the hall, or stand next to the child most likely to fail, or pass wind next to your least favourite. Unsurprisingly and disappointingly, all the teachers I've come across so far are far too busy marking and filling in Excel spreadsheets to be so inventive. Besides, the last of those games would have been an extremely risky business for me, in particular.

That's not to say life didn't feel like a live-action episode of *Bad Education* or *Teachers* from time to time. For instance, when walking down the corridor, arms full of plastic spheres sellotaped together (to demonstrate intermolecular forces), to a chime of 'Nice balls, sir!' and an outburst of giggling year ten girls. Or when urgently called outside a formally observed lesson by my friend Cesare, only for him to ask me what time we were going to the pub ('Later!'). Or when I nodded off during yet another religious assembly and the kids in my first lesson asked if I'd had a big night.

In Middlesbrough I had doors slammed in my face. In both training schools I was called all sorts, from 'Mr Tourley' and 'Mr Curly' to 'Miss Turley oops I mean Mr, hahaha' and 'Oi', 'Mate', and 'Fam'. If the kids had been paying closer attention while I

MR TOILET

was ill, a much more fitting name clearly would have been 'Mr Toilet'.

.....

When browsing Next's array of £99 suits before starting my teacher training, I was chuffed to find something original. A colour I was convinced no one else in the department would have. My mum wasn't keen but that must have been because it was just too bloomin' edgy for her to appreciate. A pseudo-maroon, chocolatey two-piece. Swaggy.

Soon after starting work striding the corridors, muffled smirks and sniggers of 'What neek[*] buys a shit-coloured suit?' suggested that maybe I should have listened to mum. But then, as it goes, if ever I didn't quite make it down that long corridor, no one would ever be able to tell! So, who was laughing really?

---

[*] A 'neek' is apparently a cross between a nerd and a geek, but I'll take it as a compliment. You need skin a good deal thicker than the cheap bog roll in staff toilets to enjoy being a teacher.

Chapter Five: Wu Wang the Poo Man

Tiger Woods came to Watford when I was ten, partly to win the World Golf Championship, but mostly to give me his autograph (I was convinced). We both wore red on matchday-Sunday, both took our fitness seriously, and both had killer short-games. And now we were both in Watford! The stars had aligned and I was off school this Friday to finally meet a fellow member of the exclusive club to which ten-year-old-me believed he belonged: legends who can make even a sport as stuffy as golf seem cool.[*]

A kids corridor was formed on the narrow walkway between the 18th green and the scoring hut. Bustling, barging boys and girls gratefully took autographs from pros, most of whom we only half-recognised. Famous faces, too, though. Phil Mickelson, Ian Poulter, all the top guys finished their rounds and spent a minimum of ten minutes working their way down with a Sharpie. Some seemed to stay almost an hour and my little red book (red to catch Tiger's attention amongst the desperate flailing arms) soon brimmed with signatures.

---

[*] See the Inbetweeners definition of golf. YouTube 'Inbetweeners Dick Faldo'.

WU WANG THE POO MAN

Excitement bristled, boiled, and then bubbled over as Tiger finally reached the last hole, a par five. His putt for an eagle 3 dropped and the crowd exploded. What a hero. That last shot ensured he had an enormous lead going into the weekend. All those other guys were good, but they weren't Tiger!

'Here he comes!'

'Tiger I love you!'

'Tiger! You the man!'

And... there he went. Not every child present was going to get his autograph, obviously. But not even one? What a bastard! Though my reduced height in the mosh would suggest otherwise, I wasn't crushed; I was pissed off. Not one! An autograph isn't even a proper signature, more of a rushed scribble, scratched onto paper in a second but etched into memory forever.

Tiger was dead to me. He won the tournament, but what's inspirational about that? It lacked any human touch and I certainly no longer shared his victories.

Maybe you think I'm being unfair. That, as an unpublished author, a failed sportsman and a 'those-who-can't' teacher, I couldn't possibly understand fame or the pressures and stresses that accompany it. Well, if you were thinking along those lines, here's my red pen: cross those lines out, because you're wrong. To prove it, let me take you to a 1,500-seat theatre on the other side of the world...

SH*T HAPPENS
Qinhuangdao, China, 2018

'Mister Jack! Mister Cesare! Miss Emma! Mister Ali! Mister Jaime!'

After an hour sweating and singing on stage there was a ten minute 'reprieve'. There was one Western toilet in the entire summer-school complex and, after jumping around for every song, I desperately needed to find it. Except, before I could, we were hounded by kids en route – they'd figured out our exit point from the stage.

They wanted selfies with puppy filters and autographs on notepads, arms, hands, toys, even a sling for one boy who'd taken a fall. They say the best time to add insult to injury is when you're signing someone's cast, but I refrained and just wrote 'Mr Jack :)'.

Given the one-minute warning pre-return to action, I finally broke free of the masses, the pain in my stomach reminding me I couldn't last another hour on stage. Promising crestfallen children who'd missed out that I'd sign later, I dashed to the loo for the world's most rushed poo. Then it was straight back to lead the crowd choreography for George Ezra's Shotgun summer tune. Then dance to Agadoo. Then Justin Bieber's Baby. Then the Macarena. I loved every second of it and the crowd could tell. Scribbling on another hand or autograph pad at the end, I was told I was no longer Mr Jack, I was 'Wu Wang', which I'm told means 'Dancing King'.

WU WANG THE POO MAN

This was singing day, and the height of the summer-camp's 1000+ attendants' euphoria at having Western teachers visit. From the moment we arrived and kids swarmed the bus, to the day we left and they stood sobbing and waving (even burly teenage boys), we visitors had a taste of what it is to be a celebrity. Lunch was more an exercise in signing autographs and answering questions in broken English than a break or time to eat. A day trip to the dragon head of the Great Wall was an extra opportunity to grab a selfie with one of us. That selfie would fast become a WeChat profile picture and soon every other kid would want an equivalent snap for their account.

Days were hot, smoggy, knackering and yet exhilaratingly rewarding. I was ill for most of the trip. Where symptoms had started to appear teaching in Gateshead and Middlesbrough, they multiplied and flourished in their new foreign environment. Imodium had saved me on many an occasion before. Now it didn't even slow things down.

The Chinese I spoke to claimed that squatting over a hole-like ground-level toilet is more hygienic than our Western, bums-on-seats method. They've clearly, clearly never had explosive diarrhoea. The toilets in the classroom block were shared with the students and only had a swinging saloon-style door which provided little to no privacy. I couldn't use those. Instead, I'd clench and waddle the three flights of stairs down, six-minute walk across the campus and one flight of stairs up to the staff-room toilets. Still just a hole in the ground and you'd better remember to bring your own bog roll.

Having the shits for a day or two is exhausting, but I'd felt rough even before we'd arrived, and things were only getting worse. I was shattered. I was tired and irritable. Grumpy and not up for anything sociable in the evenings. This wasn't me. I'd need to finally get round to seeing a doctor when I was home to get some kind of diagnosis.

A group of the staff had been to karaoke in the first week and, now a second session had been booked, I was dragged along as my new mate Jaime needed a duet partner for some Whitney Houston bangers and smash hits. To lure me out of the hotel loo, I'd been told they had a Western toilet at the karaoke club. What a treat! Ten minutes after arriving, I already needed the facilities. Ten minutes after arriving, however, instead of being treated to a homely sit on the khazi, I was clenching and sprinting back to the hotel. There was no bloody toilet paper! Do people in China have self-cleaning sphincters?!

I was at rock-plop-bottom. Back between my hotel bed and bog. Made it back to the toilet (and paper) just in time. Wiped up and now utterly wiped out. The next morning was so bad I couldn't leave the bathroom and my classes were covered. Tactically, I stopped eating at certain times of the day and made it through the rest of the trip.

WU WANG THE POO MAN

Despite telling my GP that these problems had been plaguing me before China (albeit to a lesser extent), he was convinced I'd just picked up a persistent bug in Asia and prescribed me some antibiotics. A week of them and, he assured me, I should be sorted.

.....

Having had a brief glimpse of celebrity life for a month, fun as it was, I grant Tiger that it can be energy-sapping. Perhaps I could have forgiven Eldrick Tont Woods (his real name) that day if he had been rushing to the loo. I can imagine an awkward but amusing press conference where he apologises for coming across as heartless to so many loving young fans but explains – 'When you gotta go, you gotta go.' Maybe I could have let him off the hook if he'd had a real shocker of a day, although I'm not sure. But he'd played brilliantly and, as far as anyone knows, had nothing similar to my plumbing issues. Nope, the much likelier version of events is that he was charging through the chanting, adoring crowds of children as though they weren't there because he had a hooker waiting for him in the car park.

My isolated fame was short-lived, but despite my GP's dismissive confidence, my condition wasn't. It was, in fact, incurable! Back in the summer of 2018 I still didn't have a diagnosis and, fourth course of unsuccessful antibiotics in hand, took my toileting-tour of the globe a bit closer to home. So, read on for

SH*T HAPPENS
some pain-au-chocolats, Portuguese poisons, and (as always) more painfully embarrassing poos…

Chapter Six: '*Ah, Merde*!'

Paris, France, September 2018

'Quiet please! *S'il. Vous. Plaît.*'

The jostling bustle reduces to an occasional rustle. He steps over the ball. Jittery? Shaky? Knowing that most surrounding lips are mumbling silent prayers for him to miss. But I know better than most that he doesn't care what the fans want. A perfect triangle of collarbone and hanging arms rocks the club one way, then the other. Tiger beats the ball towards the hole but, no! He's clawed it wide. A cacophonous jungle of cheers erupts; the crowd goes wild.

'OLÉ! OLÉ, OLÉ, OLÉ!'

Defiant opposition chants of 'U-S-A!' are drowned out or, better, followed up with '-can-not-play!' as

Europe edge closer to the coveted Ryder Cup.

But, *ah merde!* I shouldn't have risked that pain-au-chocolat en route to the outskirts of Paris this morning. *Le Golf National* is a huge course and while Tiger frets over a bogey (is a double-bogey one in each nostril or two-fore-one?) I have more urgent issues. I need to find *les toilettes* sharpish. We stole the word toilet from the French for 'small cloth', we even stole 'loo' from 'l'eau!', which they shouted before emptying chamber pots into the street. Searching to no avail, I had a squelching worry that we'd stolen all

SH*T HAPPENS

their actual loos along with the words. Where was the bloody bog?!

Clench and scuttle. A new walk that had already saved me on multiple occasions in the first month of my new teaching post. But, butt-problems in mind, I'd been skipping breakfast to survive mornings at work unscathed and un-skidmarked.

Why did I eat? Why today? Dad ate and I wanted to, too! Where is the sodding loo?? Clench. Scuttle. Squeeze. Clench. Just don't shit. Clench, clench, clench. I reach the brow of a hill, spot *une toilette* a few hundred yards away and mind informs useless bowel that it need not wait any longer. Ohhhhhhhhhhhhh…! Clench and scuttle deserted in a hurried flurry as I dash, desperate, towards the temporary poo-cabin. If I can just… hold… no. No, no, no. *Non! Putain! Non! Merde!*

The desperate dash becomes a downtrodden, pants-sodden dredge the last few metres. Dramatic visions of apologising as I'd burst past the queue were overly optimistic. Instead, I join the back of the line, clench, and look out for the nearest bin.

Luckily, I was wearing my best pants and the high-quality fabric made for excellent, extra-absorbent nappy material.[*] My favourite joke to tell the kids when teaching radioactivity is:

---

[*] £12 for two pairs of Calvin Kleins in TKMaxx – get on it. What a bargain!

'AH, MERDE!'

'What's the problem with Ukrainian underpants?'

'...Chernobyl fall-out!'

We teach how nuclear waste is secured in safe containers and entombed deep beneath the Earth's crust. How was I going to subtly dispose of my toxic fall-out?

Once in the cubicle I had to plot a route to smuggle my damaged goods to the bin without any of the boozed British blokes in the queue noticing. I was already drawing unwelcome attention. The duration of my sorry stay behind the door, combined with nauseating noises emanating from within, was a source of drunken toilet humour.

'Blimey someone's had a curry last night haven't they?'

'Christ, mate you can jump ahead in the queue if that one comes free first.'

Boxers mummified in a wad of loo roll, I scuttled out (no longer clenching at least) and, eyes averted from the queueing comedians, went straight to the bin. Washed my hands under the dribble and trudged back to the grassy bank where my dad sat. The crowd fell silent for another putt on the 11th green. All, except dad.

'So, you make it?'

I nodded, embarrassed enough that he'd told everyone in earshot I'd ran off to the loo, and not wishing to share the dirty details. I'd explain later. I just wanted to be back within easy reach of a nice, clean loo.

SH*T HAPPENS

I don't even like golf all that much. I'd spent a good chunk of my first month's teaching salary buying these tickets over a year ago and before 11am I was already completely wiped, exhausted, *crevé*, and going commando in some particularly chafing jeans.

.....

What was wrong with me? I still had no clue.

Multiple GP visits had only provided me with antibiotics. First, two courses for a bug picked up in China. When that didn't work, instead it was for a parasite picked up in China. Unsuccessful? Let's try another two courses of those, just in case. The antibiotics were doing nothing and my life was starting to deteriorate along with my weight and health. Meet up with friends, only to spend the whole time on the loo before a tired trek home. Hungry at work, but too shit-scared to eat.

And then there was the blood. Even when I ate minimally, I'd still be racing my bastard of a bowel to the toilet seat. No food equals no poo, surely? Sometime in September my colon decided it wanted to cough up claret too.

It didn't help that I ended up seeing a different doctor at each appointment. I must have explained the embarrassing events of the previous few months to eight different professionals now. China, Paris, sprinting out of classes when teaching up north. Admitting that Paris wasn't even the first such instance. I'd had a drink spiked in Portugal, watching football with a couple of beers and my best mate.

'AH, MERDE!'

Words slurred into poisoned slush-puppies and I slushed a great mess all over the villa floor. Back home, the race from waking up, desperate, to my toilet at the other side of the flat was one I was losing more and more often. The pile of discarded pants was growing, and my waist-line was shrinking at an alarming rate.

No medic seemed overly concerned. '75kg for your height is a healthy weight.'

'Not when I was 86kg a few weeks ago!!' (And, technically, it's not a weight but a mass. Brush up on your physics, doc.)

Eventually, after eight, nine, maybe ten GP appointments and a fair few mortifying accidents, I was granted a specialist consultation. I can only apologise to the reader for the cruder aspects of this chapter. The best way to avoid any more such stories is for us to get to the bottom of my crappy condition. And that's exactly what we'll do in Chapter Seven...

Chapter 7: Bionic Bum Fun

Hemel Hempstead Hospital, November 2018

'You have ulcerative colitis, or UC. We'll send the biopsies off to the lab to confirm.'

Never heard of it? Me neither, back in November. But after having fainted pre-procedure from either concerning consent forms, needle-nerves, or maybe just cumulative fatigue, I was glad to finally have a diagnosis. Aside from the discomfort, it was quite the experience seeing my insides via HD video; the first of an extensive al-bum the NHS would build up over the following months.

Whatever this UC was, it couldn't be too serious. A nurse pharmacist prescribed me some once-daily pills and dauntingly large enemas to pump up there every night for a couple of months until things settled. My follow-up appointment was in March. If I didn't need to see a doctor for five months it could hardly be anything life-changing. It would soon be under control and I'd be off the loo at last!

Now I had a name for it, I soon found out that a family friend's son had also been diagnosed. And a premier league footballer, and a top rugby player.

BIONIC BUM FUN

They all seemed to be doing well. At last, I was in good spirits.

Heavy sedation hadn't yet worn off. It soon did. Toilet trips returned. The first enema returned almost immediately, too. Googling to see if I should administer another, or wait for tomorrow night. Googling causes of UC: unknown. Cures for UC: unknown.

Suddenly it struck me. The pills, the escaping enemas, they were just starter drugs in a spiral of stronger and nastier medicines, none of which cured my newly identified disease. There was no cure, only management. Instead, I saw the word 'remission', which I'd only previously encountered when discussing cancer.

There was no cure? Fucking brilliant! With six-foot long, thumb-width cameras, and now added enemas, attacking my backside, not to mention countless seat-down scenarios every day, my arse was so sore it resembled the Japanese flag. But discovering all this tonight made my head hurt, too.

And there was no bloody cure. Before diagnosis, I'd never believed in crying yourself to sleep. Through previous heartbreak, or mourning, through loss; surely crying had to stop before the other could start. It wasn't just sadness, but exhaustion which finally blended the two into one. What was most knackering was accepting that this may only be the start. It took

SH*T HAPPENS

so long to arrive that I had mistaken diagnosis as the end-goal.

Eventually, it could have been at 4am, maybe 5 or 6, self-pitying sobbing soothed into that raveled sleave of care, slumber... Balm of hurt minds (and bottoms), as Macbeth famously mused.

Up. Toilet. Out, damned plop. Morning drugs. Toilet. Out, I say! Work. Loo. Hell (and toilet water) is murky. Work. Loo. Work. Home. Bog. Enema. Bog. Try to sleep. Toilet. Toilet. Toilet. Sleep. Up, toilet, and repeat.

This routine continued and worsened. Medicines were escalated as I started a course of steroids,* and briefly improved, before deteriorating even further.

An attempt at a trip to Iceland was destined to be abandoned. Moments after passing through boarding, I dashed back into the airport in desperate need. Back on the plane, landed, then an hour's drive turned into a roadside bare-bottom in sub-zero temperatures. A couple of days spent soothing my sore cheeks on a cold North Atlantic Sea seat and I resigned myself to flying home early.

I was losing blood thirty to forty times in a twenty-four-hour period. Not quite Around the World in 80 Dumps a Day, but not far from it. New Year in 2019

---

* Sadly (or maybe thankfully) not the type that supposedly make your muscles big and your penis small. Those are anabolic steroids; I was on corticosteroids.

BIONIC BUM FUN

was spent in A&E. Sent away with a higher dose of steroids. The result? No improvement whatsoever. Much like high-tech Japanese toilets, I'd resorted to hosing down my 'flag' in the shower; toilet roll becomes sandpaper when you see it every half-hour. It was hardly worth me leaving the bathroom.

I haven't written much about the pain, but it was a curl-into-foetal-position agony. Arriving in furious waves, gripping my stomach, spreading to my back. The only release was to sprint to the toilet.

By the end of the week I was finally sat before a consultant at a London hospital.

'Sometimes this disease can spiral out of control. We're going to admit you when we can find a bed tonight, put you on IV steroids. No response to that and we'll try something called rescue therapy. No response to that and I should warn you now, the last option is colorectal surgery.'

Mum had been emotional all week, but was holding it together now. Dad had held it together all week, but succumbed to rarely-breached floodgates when the doctor mentioned surgery. I was just pleased there was a plan in place. As if my next appointment was supposed to be in March... I was 86kg when I finished teacher training. On admission, I was somewhere in the high 60s. At the going rate, there wouldn't have been much left of me to take to the consultation by springtime.

SH*T HAPPENS

My first nights in hospital were punctuated by groans and screams of anguish I'd hoped would never be mine. They weren't yet, but they soon would be. There was an elderly Jamaican man, clearly in agony, fuming at the nurses, doctors, and the world. Old-age always petrified me to ponder, with its promise of loss, dependence, and decline. Death and illness were inconvenient realities I'd prefer to keep at bay.

Perhaps this is why I like working with young people. In schools, life bursts with the strongest and best of emotions. I tried an office job and could detect days drifting and dying into nothing all too soon. Doctors, nurses – they have a mindset I can only admire, yet not quite comprehend. They directly combat death, misery and tragedy, and the worst of emotions, on a daily basis.

Nurses face the brunt of the drama on the ward. The angry patients, suffering patients, impatient patients and the confused ones. The posh* prat who mistakes St Thomas' for the Marriott Hotel, which neighbours the hospital along the Thames. Or the guy whose girlfriend proclaims 'Bruv, hehehe, put your penis away! Dere's people dyin' in here!'

---

* I recently discovered via my wise ol' grandad that the word 'posh' stems from 'Port Out, Starboard, Home'; the side of a cruise liner which would have the sun for each leg of the journey between England and India back int' day.

BIONIC BUM FUN

Or even the bloke who blares Jeremy Kyle from his bedside screen (why couldn't it have been cancelled before I was admitted??), but makes up for it by offering around snacks stolen from the M&S downstairs.

Five days of intravenous steroid injections every few hours achieved nothing. They did succeed in bloating my face and brittling my joints, but the symptoms were as toilet terrible as ever.

Time for rescue therapy: an old form of chemotherapy found to be better for Crohn's and colitis than for the big C. There's a list of side effects longer than my large intestine for this drug, called Infliximab. During my first infusion I was meant to be checked every fifteen minutes. Linked up to the drip-machine, administration would last two hours. But then, disaster struck. My nurse went for lunch, and the assistant tasked with my monitoring a) only paid one visit in the first hour and b) didn't have the slightest idea what to do when I was curled up, groaning in the foetal position, desperate for a toilet trip. Could we unplug the machine providing the infusion? It beeped madly when she tried.

I begged for a bed-pan but the assistant scrunched her nose and admonished, 'Oh you don't want to do that.' She was ignorant to my pain and oblivious to the very real risk I'd make a mess much further-reaching than a bed-pan if I didn't get to the bathroom right away. Her solution was to unplug the drip for a few minutes while I dashed to the loo. It was all guesswork. Didn't she get it?! This was rescue therapy. And I wanted to be rescued! It's well worth crapping in a cardboard cup to be rescued! Luckily, after the nurse returned, she recognised a faulty battery in the machine and switched that so I could unplug and release the pain freely for the last forty-five minutes.

That night, I was moved from Nightinhell Ward to the gastro-specific treatment ward. Finally, I felt in good hands. Over the weekend, the therapy kicked in and the following week, I was a free man, and just in time for my birthday!

The rescue therapy is designed to last eight weeks per infusion. Within eight days I was back in hospital, where an advanced second dose showed no response, and no rescue. So that was it, last resort: chop out the faulty bits – namely the entirety of my large intestine. I had exhausted the full repertoire of medicinal options the NHS offers and it was time to meet the surgeon each morning on the ward, instead of the gastro-medicinal team.

A stoma nurse came to see me to discuss how having an arse in my abs would change my life, and to ascertain where specifically on my abdomen I'd like this new orifice. I didn't care about the aesthetics, I just wanted the bag as far away from my business as feasible. I'd read a delightful article online about it sounding like a crisp packet slapping between two bodies. As much as I do bloody love crisps, I'd prefer not to have a packet in my pocket during life's more intimate moments.

But then, before what would have been one of the last meetings with the doctors on the medication side of affairs, I was given some industry insight – a beacon of hope, from a lovely pair of elderly Sheilas.[*] They had spotted in the newspaper a piece on a new drug for UC and they both cut out the same article for me, just in time, too. It was called Tofacitinib and wasn't yet fully licensed across the UK, but after initially poo-pooing its chances of stopping me from doing exactly that, the team decided it was worth a try.

Having never been great with swallowing pills, I choked on the first dose after the nurse branded me a wuss for asking to crush it. After clarifying that crushing it was, in fact, a better idea from now on, and cleaning up the puddle of curry that had come up all over the visitors' room along with the pill projectile, I went to bed. Over the weekend, the new drug kicked in and the following week, I was a free man, and not just for eight days this time.

This was February. Steroids had taken a profound effect on my body. At its worst, my joints were brittle to the point I required assistance just to get from bed to bathroom. Steroids never allow you to sleep much,

---

[*] One was my nan; one was my ex's; both were called Sheila. I'm indebted to them both for their efforts in reading the Daily Mail. I could never do it.

but as soon as the intestinal agony had gone, the joint pain arrived to keep me awake all night. I stayed at my parents' rather than returning to my flat. Mum left my door open so if the standard groans morphed into something worse, she could come. Or if I needed the toilet, or more painkillers. Being so incapacitated was frustrating beyond belief. Guilt and impatience filled any rare moments of reprieve from the physical pain.

As I switched from IV to oral steroids and began a slow wean from these dirtiest of drugs, the side effects began to reside. I was back at work by March to polite, if intrusive, inquisitions from pupils of 'Sir, what's happened to your face?' or later, 'You look a bit less inflated this week, Sir.' To match the water-weight retained on my face, I had man-boobs, back-blubbers and kankles – stood in contrast to my emaciated muscles. Looking in the mirror, I was unable to recognise the sorry figure scowling back at me with sunken eyes. I bumped into the mum of an old friend. She knew me well from age eight to eighteen. We chatted with an unusual unfamiliarity for a minute before finally she asked who I was. She hid her shock graciously.

As spring became summer, I neared the end of my seven-month, abusive, love-hate relationship with steroids. Everyone at work, staff, pupils, friends outside, commented on how much better I was looking. The issue was hidden. Ulcerative colitis is an invisible illness (providing you don't log my loo-data)

BIONIC BUM FUN

and to truly be 'better', I needed Tofacitinib to work without steroids propping me up. Within a couple of weeks of breaking up with steroids, I was back in hospital – back at square-one.

The next two weeks whizz by in a hazy, unhappy flurry of drugs, consultations, and acceptance that surgery was the only route out of the disease. Ulcerative colitis also has no known cure, but as I said at the beginning of this toilet trip we've taken together, body minus colon equals no colitis.

I told friends how long the surgery could be to responses of 'Can't believe you're going to be under the knife for nine hours!', 'So you're never going to be able to fart again?!?', and 'Are you going to be put out for that whole time?'

All I could reply was, 'I bloody well hope so!' Another, more understanding, friend, who had undergone a similar surgery at the start of the year, told me the epidural insertion was the worst part. But it would only take a few minutes and then I'd be off my rocker on opiates upon waking up. The fact that it took around half an hour to successfully fit the epidural really should have warned me not to expect a smooth transition on the other side.

However, this brings us back to where we started in Chapter One, and so we conclude our crude tour of the globe. In the three months since I escaped hospital, I've still had pain on many days. But it's becoming less frequent as I recover. I have a minimum of one more major surgery to come. But I don't need to think about that for now, so I won't.

I've woken up in a tent, covered in you-know-what, and brushed it through my best mate's hair trying to find tissues and a torch in the dark. But then, Sh*t Happens!

On the sunnier side, I've also returned full-time to the job I love and have been accepted for additional work with vulnerable children, something I would never have had the energy to commit to when fighting daily battles with this absolute minger of a disease.

More recently, I've even played some tennis, been pissed in Poland, climbed a mountain, regained most of the weight I lost and reconnected with friends with whom I was too zombie-like to socialise for over a year. I look in the mirror and, yes, where there could be a half-decent set of abs there is, instead, an arse. Sexy! But that sort of thing means very little. Consumed by illness and gone for over a year, I'm once again looking at a version of myself I recognise.

Thank you to everyone who has read, half-read, or got in touch; I hope you've enjoyed the journey! Writing has been an anchor tethering me to my sanity throughout this shit-storm of a disease; it's been brilliant to hear people say that reading this has, in some small way, helped them deal with their own mental or physical struggles.

But an anchor alone won't help escape the storm; humour has been both the boat and paddle by which

BIONIC BUM FUN

I've left this rough time behind me and escaped Shit Creek. Sharing humour with family and friends reinforces that boat, ready for future choppy waters. Now, I'll let you get back to what you were doing, and I'm off to do something that doesn't involve sitting on the loo!*

---

* How optimistic…

Series (Number) Two

Chapter One: Same Sh*t, Different Surgery

St Thomas' Hospital, London, September 2020

Seven hours until I'll have my action man ass fitted and, once again, there's little hope of sleep. Back in St Thomas' hospital, I've avoided Nightinhell Ward. This time, I'm locked down (rather fittingly) in Northumberland Ward. The view of the London Eye, Thames, and Charing Cross Station was as terrific as it was brief, before the window-side bed occupants pulled their curtains, shutting the world off for me.

Groans of pain still emanate from the diagonally opposite bed. The old boy two metres to my right has a new colostomy and his surgery gas is deflating in whoopie cushion thunders. In another bay, out of sight, someone's drip feed has run out and will beep, beep, beep until the night nurse has time to attend to it. My machine realises that it, too, is low on battery and subsequently chimes in beeping unison.

Daylight hours aren't any calmer, since the day room is having raucous roof and wall repairs. The rest of the world is eleven floors downstairs. Family and friends, who kept me laughing through all the weeks

SAME SH*T, DIFFERENT SURGERY

stuck here in 2019, feel infinitely more distant through a screen.

The gap between my first op and tomorrow's could have been fifteen years, all things being well. Beep. I didn't even manage fifteen months. This fucking beeping is enough to drive anyone mental.

Let's talk about something more fun. I know sequels are expected to be shit, but I don't want to plop too heavy, too soon. We'll save the sticky subjects like mental health for another day. So, we'll ease into this second series with a few farting fables…

Ostomy bags can stick straight over your stoma onto the skin (a one-piece system) or the bag can clip onto a plaster-like adhesive square (a two-piece). I don't tell the stoma nurse why I insist on a two-piece system. And so you might wonder 'What is the embarrassing reason behind this?' If this is anything like the Sh*t Happens of old, is it sex related? Or another naked Latvian man?! Saucy!

Nope. The answer is, of course, farting. Which isn't nearly as juicy, unless you're doing your flatulence very wrong indeed.

In an average twenty-four hours, I empty the stoma bag once around 4am, and then maybe five times between morning and night. Six trips might already seem like a pain in the artificial arse to deal with. But that number could be significantly higher still, if it wasn't for that most basic of human instincts, passing wind.

SH*T HAPPENS

I thought my fun-filled days of flatulence were over when I lost my large bowel to ulcerative colitis. Turns out, I can still fart! But only with a two-piece – and this is the key. If the bag balloons, ready to pop, then sneaking a silent-but-violent is as simple as briefly unclipping the top of the bag and letting some gas escape. Doing so every day saves a trip or two to the loo. Clever, eh?

Kelly Forest, Kent, September 2019

Two months after my last surgery, I was getting to grips with how the stoma functions. My confidence had grown to the point that when a mate suggested an impromptu camping trip, this felt like the closest thing to a holiday I'd had in a long time. Why let the bears and popes have all the fun digging trenches in the woods?

Anyway, after a barbecue and a few cans of Guinness,* the three of us were drunkenly dropping off in the pitch black of the tent. I lay in the middle. Between me and the entrance I had my flatmate (and best mate), commonly known as the Rake.

Spatters of rain and wind billowing at the tent told me the weather had turned, but my overworked digestive system didn't care. The bag started to bulge.

---

* Check out my appearance on The After Hours Lounge (Spotify/Apple Podcasts) to hear me chatting shit about Guinness, tennis, and mental health.

SAME SH*T, DIFFERENT SURGERY

I really couldn't be bothered to move, let alone traipse out into the dark and damp to unload.

But, aha! Luckily, I had the two-piece system. A good ol' fashioned puff should provide a buffer to see me through until sunrise.

It's important to realise that, during my two years of consistent illness and irregular socialising, any previous alcohol tolerance had dropped to almost-Mormon levels. Despite making a living teaching physics, I suffered a brief lapse in my understanding of basic gravity. Lying on my back, I went for a cheeky unclip-and-release. My friends were passed out by now anyway, so they wouldn't catch a whiff.

Alas, gravity sobered me up instantaneously, as oozing contents warmed my stomach and chest, the situation becoming stickier (and this story juicier) than I'd ever hoped.

'Ah, sh*t!'

Neither friend stirred. Frantically, I searched for the end of the duffel bag I had been using as a pillow. There were spare bags and tissues in there. In the pooey panic and absence of light, I'd completely lost my bearings. My gruesome, groping hands brushed across something… but it wasn't my holdall. It was my best mate's head. Somehow, the Rake didn't wake.

Torch, bag, and tissues located, I clambered over the poorly placed Rake, out of the tent and fumbled the shoddiest bag change I've yet managed, using a

SH*T HAPPENS

near empty bottle of hand-san and our drinking water to clean up.

Both friends remained passed out, pre-hangover. So, I decided to save the dirty details until we were within reach of running water the next day. Learning the truth twenty hours later, Rake took it, unsurprisingly, admirably well. Outside of family, no one was there for me more than him through the torrid toilet times. So, he was best prepared for some follow-up follow-through, after all.

.....

Writing this has dragged me closer to surgery number two. In a few long hours, my rectum will be removed, and my retracted stoma refashioned into its original form. I'll be sewn up at both the front and back. If there was a god, I'd be praying for less pain this time around. But my agonal cries certainly weren't heard in 2018, or 2019. So, I won't yet pin my hopes on 2020 being any better. As Stephen Fry famously said: "Why should I respect a capricious, mean-minded, stupid god who creates a world that is so full of injustice and pain?"[*]

After plumbing the depths of my earlier tales, this one may have felt like all fart and no poo (or rather, just a little bit of poo). I've only really skid-marked the surface here, but Sh*t Keeps Happening, and I can assure you the next chapter promises to be a squelcher.

---

[*] YouTube 'Stephen Fry on God'.

Chapter Two: Lost the Plop

Upgraded to the window bed, I'm taking in London from eleven floors up and hoping I'm not back anytime soon. Knowing I've got this stoma for the next eighty-odd years, I'll likely be back from time to time.

No one mentioned before my first op, for example, that seventy percent of stoma patients go on to develop hernias or peristomal hernias at some point in their lives. And I've got longer than most for delightful shit like that to occur.

The friendly guys in their 50s and 60s having similar bowel and rectal surgeries for cancer all managed to escape a couple of days before me. They joked I was the last of the musketeers.

Their replacements are less chatty. A Jamaican man in his 80s sits staring emptily into nothing. I know his name is Roy and I try to strike up some small talk when passing for the toilet. But he offers no verbal response, hardly any recognition at all, and the only noise ever reaching me from the old fella are his mumbled prayers before sleep (or attempts to sleep, if he's anything like me).

SH*T HAPPENS

Those of you who have read *Causa** may know the opening was, in part, inspired by the death of my uncle, John, a former navy man. Although I was too young to fully grasp the reasons behind his suicide at the time, I know he had a real fear of ending up stuck in hospital for the remainder of his days. Instead, he chose to end things on his terms, in the sea.

In quiet moments, I question my resilience to this condition further down the line. After countless outpatient appointments in 2018 and then four lengthy admissions in 2019, the February news that I would be back for further surgery this year arrived with a disproportionate sense of dread.

The surgery was necessary, but it seemed all too soon. Ten or fifteen bloody years too soon. Physically, I went into this operation in significantly better shape than the last one. Mentally, however, it only felt as though I was only just recovering, and now I was being flung right back into where the poo splatters the fan.

This initial dread simmered and settled, revealing itself in uncharacteristic bursts of anger. Here are a few examples of when I lost the plot, since having lost the ability to plop. Hope you enjoy!

---

* My debut novel – set across Brazil, Britain, and Russia.

LOST THE PLOP
Lockdown, St Albans, 2020

This year I've exploded with a frequency and unpredictability that frightens me. Previously, I'd seen the so-called 'Turley Temper' as a positive, because I'd channel it and I was in control. It helped me battle to tennis victories, ensured I never took shit from anyone as a kid, and got fired up to stand up for people and causes I cared about.

A few years back, a particularly officious tennis referee made my mum cry at junior nationals after she informed him that we couldn't afford to stay solely for the doubles. My blood scalded, vaporising between my ears, but I harnessed that anger to do the right thing and made the bullying gammon of a man feel the fool.

Inherited from my dad, I'd seen this temper protect the ones he loved when, in its absence, they would have been downtrodden.

Recently though, that rare, proud temper has morphed into an aimless, regular hindrance. I broke a tennis racket in training (something I'm not known for doing even in matches), upturned tables and chairs in my flat (just, why?), and lost my rag for all sorts of menial troubles.

A formerly very close friend of mine helped royally trash my car in 2019, causing over £500 of damage to an '04 plate Yaris that simply isn't worth spending that much money on. After he refused to offer any remorse – let alone financial assistance – in sorting it out, I thought, 'Well, fuck him' and carried on merrily with my life.

After discovering I was back for the chop, however, sighting the unfixed dents in my grandad's old car ignited a fury far more livid than I had experienced at the time of the incident. Months on from the mishap, disgruntlement boiled and spluttered each time I remembered and, on a few occasions, I found myself kicking the bumps in the car. The car! What did the poor Yaris do? Its number plate ends in BLV – standing for Bloody Lovely Vehicle – and it certainly deserves better than it gets from both me and my mates.

In lockdown, we've been very fortunate that our flat has a small private garden and, while tennis courts were off-limits, had a table tennis table for staying sharp. Over the course of 2020, I broke three bats! Three! And dealing with my outbursts must have rubbed off on my girlfriend because she ended up throwing a bat so hard it flew through a hedge and into the neighbour's garden.

Luckily, I used everything learnt from SAS man Mark 'Billy' Billingham's autobiography *The Hard Way* and retrieved the bat in a covert operation. Feigning a lost ball, I rummaged around in the dear old girl in the flat below's bush, then emerged brandishing a ball (smuggled in with me), discreetly having pinched the bat.

And before you get excited with a smart quip about me and an elderly resident's bush, you can find

LOST THE PLOP

a wholesome picture of me trimming the hedge in question on Instagram.

In all seriousness, I'm hoping that the last few months of uncharacteristic anger are nothing more than a blip. I'm putting it down to stress. Sitting on the knowledge that a surgeon will soon cut out what you're sitting on doesn't make for comfortable sitting.*

Other than my girlfriend, who has tirelessly and lovingly endured my quasi-bipolar nature throughout the virus situation, I wonder if many of my friends and family will have noticed any change at all. Although I say these spates of fury feel uncontrollable, they only appear to reside in my private life. Both my social and professional lives are spared any creeping nuisance.

This is what I referred to when writing about the 'side you don't see' for world suicide prevention day. If a close one seems a bit 'off', maybe they are. People don't just suddenly change and shut off from the world for no good reason.

My uncle's fear was being trapped in a hospital. My similar apprehension manifested in outbursts of rage.

Since writing the start of this chapter, I've followed the other musketeers and escaped the hospital. Hopefully, this signals a new chapter for the Turley Temper as it returns quietly to the bench, only

---

* Say 'sitting' more, I know!

subbing on when summoned by the manager. You can check my bank statements for table tennis bat purchases in a few months to see if I've tamed the beast.

For now, I'm off to think about the next big challenge: learning to sit in a chair without it being (quite literally) a massive pain in the arse. Until next time!

Chapter Three: Loo-ful Meditation

Stress levels skyrocketed in the build-up to my recent surgery. It got so bad, I even tried meditation. I know, *meditation* - blimey.

Facing a non-negligible chance your 'business' won't work after an op certainly raises the stakes. As I've said, the surgeon's registrar informed me they *had* hoped to avoid this surgery for at least a decade, leaving plenty of time for enjoying sex (and ideally to have a family). The numbers varied with who I spoke to, but the general gist was the impotency rates could be as high as ten percent.

Ulcerative colitis intervened a mere few months into those potential fifteen years, determined as ever to wreck me. Attempts to calm my inflamed rectum with drugs only resulted in more escaping enemas and bloody messes.

Now, you might think the risk is pretty small. 'Think positive,' you say. Plenty of my mates attempted reassurance, citing the ninety percent probability of no damage. Nevertheless, if any of them were given a pack of ten skittles and told one would stop their penis functioning, I'm fairly sure they'd leave the fucking skittles alone!

Thankfully, the all-important nerves survived the procedure.

SH*T HAPPENS

And I haven't meditated since. Science says it has a lot of benefits, I'm aware. But I just felt like such a plonker sitting there trying it. A sore wound where my anus used to be, even resting on a chair is a pain in the action man arse at the minute. So, I'll place the lotus position to one side, with a tentative note to try again in the future.

Pooing, I believe, is a man's preferred and most widely accepted form of meditation. Doctors have explained the relaxing effect of taking a dump,* and men seem to spend more time on the bog than women. When facing mockery for trying other more public forms of meditation, why waste such a zen moment by rushing back out into the world?

As a kid I would leave books in different toilets. So, while I might be reading Harry Potter in bed, the Cherub action series would entertain trips to the family bathroom and maybe *Zombie Bums From Uranus* occupied the loo over at my grandad's. Born ten years later, I may have just scrolled social media. I'm glad that wasn't the case – I'd have been missing out.

---

* Google it next time you're sitting on the throne (assuming that's not where you're reading this, in which case feel free to read on).

LOO-FUL MEDITATION
St Thomas' and St Albans, 2020

Waking up with no bum was less traumatic than coming-to with no colon. Last time, my pain relief epidural dislodged, and I regained consciousness screaming in anguish, like the Darkseeker Will Smith chains to the bed in *I Am Legend*.

With this recent surgery, I woke up woozy but chatty. I vaguely remember speaking about Sh*t Happens to a nurse and this memory was confirmed when she left a comment on the J E Turley website a few days later.

The worst pain experienced during this visit was having a drain removed from my backside wound. If those vulnerable nerves had survived the main procedure, then it felt as though they were being hacked through with a chainsaw as the nurse slowly extracted the tube. I screamed like a little Turl for the duration of the encounter.

One of the frustrating aspects of having an ileostomy is the time spent throughout the day (and night) emptying or changing the bag. Whereas a standard zen men's moment in the bog is a hands-free, sit and relax, my new loo routine is hands-on and hunched over. Hardly an opportunity to unwind. And no chance to get lost in a good book.

Or so I thought, until I started listening to audiobooks whenever dealing with the bag. My hands may be occupied, but my ears and mind are free for a story. Meditative toilet trips were back, and mindful moments sat on the loo lived to last another day.

Even now that I have my barbie bum, I still might have a feasible excuse to sit on the toilet: the 'phantom rectum'.

The human brain struggles to adjust to a severed limb and saying goodbye to your bottom is no different. Those missing an arm or a leg often suffer from an itch on the limb that isn't there – the so-called phantom limb – which is usually best-solved by clever use of mirrors to mimic the missing body part.

With a phantom rectum, mirrors aren't much use. So far, I've experienced unpredictable bursts of agony. Minding my own business, the phantom menace strikes, and it is as though a piranha has jumped out of thin air to bite me in the behind.

The phantom rectum can also manifest in an urge to go to the toilet the old-fashioned (and now impossible) way, or as an itch that just won't bog off. Except, strangely enough, 'bogging' off can be exactly the remedy. Sitting on the loo and play-acting can help flush away the phantom.

So, there you have it. The many marvellous benefits of loo-full meditation apply whatever the state of your arse.

LOO-FUL MEDITATION

Next time, we take our final trip along the pooey path of Sh*t Happens and, I hope, will (skid-)mark the end to this whole messy business.*

---

* You might have spotted I've dropped the 'Around the World in 80 Dumps a Day' title for this series. The coronavirus (and being an at-risk person) has ensured recent sh*t only happened in the UK.

Chapter Four: The Final Flush

Try as I may, it's hard to consider a positive spin,
For a deathly disease, leaving me weak, and thin.

At last. It's all over.

The disease has gone. Incinerated along with my colon, rectum, and the foolish, hopeful sense of invincibility I once carried.

Back teaching, I'm also now running a lecture club, the Stephen Hawking Society, named after the school's most famous alumnus.

Having read (most of) *A Brief History of Time* and (all of) *Brief Answers to the Big Questions*, I have a passable understanding of the great thinker's physics. I realised, though, that I knew very little about his personal and medical journey. Keen to rectify this, I watched *The Theory of Everything*, which is based on a book by Hawking's first wife, Jane, called *Travelling to Infinity: My Life with Stephen*.

The film is as devastating as it is inspiring. A rising lump constantly threatened to swell and clog my throat throughout. It reached its most severe inflammation in the aftermath of Hawking's diagnosis, when Eddie Redmayne says: 'You don't understand. This is going to affect everything.'

THE FINAL FLUSH

Now, the difference between what Hawking faced with motor neurone disease compared with ulcerative colitis is as vast as the gulf between our respective understandings of cosmology, but the poignancy of the quote resonated with me.

It hit me because of the tragedy of their romance, his world upended just a year after meeting Jane. And the lump became too sizeable to gulp down because of its parallels with my universe.

London and St Albans, 2019–20

A lot happened in my first 193 days without a colon. If you've read this far, you'll know all about the shit shenanigans. But it wasn't all crap. I'd met a girl, for one. Tatiana, or T.

The first time she ventured to stay at mine, my stoma decided to carry out a character judgement. Walking back from the station, the bag suddenly felt very full, and especially weighty. We'd had a liquid dinner, dancing and smiling, storytelling and joking, so I was surprised at how heavy the contents felt.

It needn't cause concern. I'd let T freshen up and then sort my 'belly' out. Tipsily setting myself down on the loo, I opened the Velcro folds at the base of the bag and, perplexingly, nothing came out. Gravity sometimes needs assistance, so I squeezed the contents of the bag, guiding them down and out. Still, nothing. I had opened the bag, hadn't I?

SH*T HAPPENS

T is Russian and had drunk me under the table, but I wasn't so far gone that I had forgotten any glaringly obvious part of my new pooing procedure. I squeezed a little harder and felt a tug on my abdomen.

And then, emerging from a haze of romance, excitement, and vodka-induced serenity, reality suddenly hit me. The stoma has no nerve endings. I was squeezing my small fucking intestine!

I frantically removed the bag and fuck fuck fuck fuck fuck fuck fuck fuck fuck fuck fuck fuck fuck.

Fuck.

My stoma had prolapsed and a girthy six inches[*] of intestine was hanging out from my abdomen. I'd seen it temporarily retract below the surface of my skin a couple of times before, and it's natural for the bowel to move a small amount, but this was on another, more gruesome, level.

I'd been gone a while now and T was knocking on the door, checking I hadn't fallen in the loo. Fuck. It would've been easier to explain if I had.

'Won't be a minute!' I replied, wishing I sounded suave, but instead coming across scared. 'Just a little problem, won't be a mo.'

I replaced the bag and came out, defeated. I explained to T what was happening and tried to act less concerned than I felt. Any further fun was off the cards.

---

[*] Title of my sex tape…

THE FINAL FLUSH

She was completely understanding, reassuring, and suggested we go to A&E. I wanted to give it an hour or so to see if the stoma retracted at all by itself. T fell asleep and forty-five minutes later, the stoma and I agreed she had aced his character test, and he decided to shrivel down to his own slumber.

4 February, 2020

After the first major surgery in July '19, a follow-up appointment with my surgeon should have taken place six to eight weeks into recovery. Somehow, I slipped through the NHS booking system on multiple occasions. The checkup finally happened almost six months later.

By now, we'd been dating a couple of months and T had dropped enough hints about still being 'single' that I wanted to ask her out properly. Inconveniently, I was working abroad on Valentine's Day. Well, that is if you can class drinking port and cheering on FC Porto on the school football tour as 'work'.

During these first weeks of 2020 I was thrilled beyond belief, just relieved to finally be back living life unchained from the loo. However, in the absence of a follow-up appointment with the surgeon, I was also pretending everything was running smoothly with my health. It wasn't.

Despite no longer serving any functional purpose, my rectum was still ravaged by the disease. Although the urgency was largely gone, I still lost blood during a handful of toilet trips each day. To make matters worse, my stoma had now permanently retracted beneath the surrounding skin, meaning waste in effect just forced its way out of my abdomen. Excruciating pain ensued; a sensation akin to a Bunsen burner flame held to my skin almost incessantly. With the stoma hidden, leakages were a constant threat and pain, once again, returned as an accepted, albeit depressing, part of the everyday routine.

The surgeon informed me he could operate as soon as March. They would remove my rectum and refashion the stoma. (As if it ever went out of fashion!) With another major surgery inevitable, I was determined to finish my already interrupted and delayed year as a Newly Qualified Teacher and asked if we could postpone action until July (which Covid ultimately pushed back to September). Avoiding the slog of NQT paperwork for a further year was worth a few extra months of stoma complications.

After my appointment, I'd planned to see T and maybe give her the envelope titled 'Not to be opened before 14 February' (and yes, alright, I'll admit it contained a poem).

Instead, I arrived at her flat trying to hide just how distraught I was. It was the start of what was a prolonged period of angst at the thought of going through the whole ordeal again.

On 4 February, 193 days on from my surgery, I asked myself 'Why *now*?' Why, having just met

THE FINAL FLUSH

someone, was I going to be forced to do it all once again? As with diagnosis, it felt too fucking soon.

By no means did I wish to abandon hope for this relationship, but I was wracked with guilt already, and I hadn't even asked her to be my bloody girlfriend yet. Other than on that evening after the appointment, I think I managed to conceal it from T pretty well. It was too early in a relationship to share such a burden.

But then Covid happened, and just a few weeks after becoming 'official' (not Facebook official, though, too soon for that big step clearly) I asked her if she'd like to spend lockdown at my flat, along with her cats. Rushed as that may seem, neither of us wanted a Zoom call relationship.

This was great, and a decision I'll never regret (and not just because I adore little Ivy and Lio). But it also meant T was exposed to a side of me I'd hoped she'd never need to see.

Romance was tested immediately with nightly steroid enemas intruding (quite literally) in the bedroom. Nighttime leaks, gushing blood, and even T finding me collapsed on the floor mid bag change, calling out for help and catching the splurting contents with a cupped hand. I was reduced to a hopeless, pathetic patient; hardly the charming romantic prospect I aspired to be. This is a side friends and family don't often see, a side I didn't wish to impose on anyone, least of all my gorgeous girlfriend. Just as I couldn't believe my luck to have met her, faced so soon as she was with all this, I thought she must surely be cursing hers.

This was the outset of a settling dread. A dark cloud blanketing into post-volcanic ash, it clogged my every thought, fear, and mood. It showed no signs of clearing until the operation passed.

One reason I was so gutted (pardon the cheap pun but I'm running out by now) is that, excited as I was to meet T, I almost wished it could have happened a year later. I was scared the illness would affect everything, poison everything, our fledgling relationship included. This may sound defeatist, but my long battle with the disease has taught me that ulcerative colitis does just that.

Hawking understood this concept. But I don't think those untouched by medical misfortune can fully grasp it. I hope Sh*t Happens has entertained – that was my goal, after all, starting out. However, while a lot of my experiences have been amusing, a vanishingly small proportion of having a chronic illness is, in reality, even remotely fun.

If my physical fitness was severely diminished by the disease, then my mental fortitude was completely obliterated. My confidence hit rock bottom. I became insecure, a shell of my usual, smiling character and hard to be around. Crippled with self-doubt, I feared fulfilling my gloomy prophecy for our relationship, and in doing so I had brought a negative outcome closer.

THE FINAL FLUSH

In short, I was miserable and scared – a hollowed-out ruin in place of my former mojo. I tried and failed to remember the confident guy who chatted to T at the tennis tournament where we'd met. Distant already, it was all a forgotten show, with a stage as rotten as my insides.

Both Stephen Hawking and Jane were thrown into bouts of depression in confronting his illness. Stephen, in particular, used humour to overcome the darkness. Humour, and work. In cosmology, he found a passion and stuck at it until his death, saying, 'however difficult life may seem, there is always something you can do and succeed at' and 'work gives you meaning and purpose and life is empty without it'.

Writing has been both my work and my purpose. Since diagnosis, I've written a novel (*Causa*), started a second (*Billions and One*), and had countless articles published. At times I don't feel particularly inspired (sitting on the loo led to *Sh*t Happens*, but some days I guess it's less awe inspiring) and in those moments I might just jot down a few thoughts. It helps declutter my mind and flush away all the unwanted confusion. There have been moments where I'd look back on old goals young-me once set. I mourn that version of me, happily shitting from my arse and not appreciating life's functional simplicity. But I also look at more recent goals and can appreciate how far I've come from the sorry figure I cut in Chapter Two, staring at my wrists and wondering when it might all finally be over.

It is over, now, but not like that.

The medications are over. The uncertainty is over. The urgency, gone. And I can't have any more majorly major surgeries since they've chopped out everything that was dodgy. My family and friends got me through my first surgery. The nature of Covid and isolation has meant that T had to get me through the second one on her own. She was so lovely throughout; if only I was better at physics then maybe she could have got a film made out of it. *The Theory of Shitting* doesn't really have a ring to it, though, unfortunately.

I left her alone in tears on her 25th birthday as I was taken in for surgery on 17 September. The video of messages from all my loved ones, which she pieced together, would have made me cry, too, if I hadn't dozed off the first three times I tried to watch it. I was still pretty drugged up, clearly – not a reflection on the video at all; it was amazing. Those were rough days. Now, as 2020 finally comes to a close, I think we may at last be paddling beyond shit creek.

Yes, there are still downsides to having a stoma bag.

And there are a few things I can no longer do. Going to Nando's and not getting a corn on the cob is miserable. Knackered, wanting to fall asleep after a long day but needing to sort the bag out is an inconvenience and is draining, mentally. Getting

THE FINAL FLUSH

fresh out the shower, removing an old bag and the stoma shitting down my leg before I can replace it is never an ideal way to start a Monday, but also not all that uncommon.

After a couple of months pain free, I had my follow-up appointments with both the surgeon and stoma nurse mid-way through writing this chapter. The surgeon said that, providing nothing goes wrong this time, he shouldn't need to see me again. I thanked him for giving me my life back and hoped that would be our last conversation. The stoma nurses were happy with my bag system and pencilled me in for a check-up six months down the line.

Alas, nothing is ever straightforward with this disease and within days of those meetings, complications have crept back into my day. The stoma has, once again, retracted beneath the surface of my abdomen. On cue, pain and renewed leakages followed. Late last night, I googled 'retracted stoma' and confirmed my fear that surgery might, once again, be necessary if the problems persist. One article offered the following ridiculous truism as advice: 'The most effective method of preventing a stoma complication is avoiding the creation of a stoma.'

Reading this, the dread of persistent pain rushed back to me and I lost the plot. As a result, I am typing this up with two extremely sore hands, a wall that needs replastering and a demolished clothes dryer, wrangled beyond repair. I can only apologise to T

SH*T HAPPENS

and, more importantly, the cats for frightening them with my outbursts.

I slept for almost twelve hours last night. Not because I was especially tired physically, nor because it's Christmas at the time of writing and in tier four Covid restrictions there's little else to do, but because I didn't want to face another surgery. This disease is a monstrous bastard to deal with. If there really is a god – a god who made colitis and coronavirus and cancer and Crohn's (plus all the other illnesses that don't start with 'c') – well, I think that god is a cunt.*

But I want to conclude on a positive note. I'm not finding it all that easy, clearly. Perhaps looking back on some low points, and I mean the *real* lows, might help. Equally, it could just make things worse. Only one way to find out:

Shuffling to the toilet with crippled stature. Falling from the edge of my hospital bed into the window as my knees lost the ability to carry my weight. Arms bruised, sucked, and pinched purple, worse than any junkie. Shitting on a cold highway in Iceland. Shitting myself in Paris. Shitting myself at all! Long, lonely nights and, incapacitated, days slipping away into an extended nothing…

'All the world's a stage,

And all the men and women merely players.'

---

* Sorry if that offended anyone but if you were that pious you wouldn't have made it to the final chapter of a book titled Sh*t Happens, so deal with it.

THE FINAL FLUSH

This Shakespeare quote stayed with me. It opens the description of the Seven Ages of Man. Meeting T, I should have been at the third stage, the lover. Instead, the disease does its best to beat me into 'mere oblivion', the final stage, 'sans everything'.

Joints in agony, advanced ageing. Face bloated. Body itching. Sleep a distant memory. Memory, itself, opaquely foggy. Stomach twisted, in tatters. Arse a wreck. Emotions all encompassing. Death – all that awaits beyond the seventh stage – suddenly tangible, seemingly close enough to touch; and not frightening (as I'd always assumed), but welcoming, at last an unending reprieve from the inescapable suffering.

Remembering such depths of despair, the present moment doesn't seem too bad, after all. Put in perspective, that post-shower bag change isn't too unwieldy a task. That restrictive hernia belt is hardly the end of the world. Getting up once a night for toilet trips is better than fearing every fart and writhing on the floor in torturous pain. And worrying about weird-looking abs is far, far easier than wishing away my life.

With the stoma, I'm in control. It might cause me pain, and it could lead to further surgeries, but I've survived them before, and I'd get through them again. The second operation wasn't as traumatic as the first. A third wouldn't be a socially distanced walk in the park, but I now know I would manage.

Around the World in 80 Dumps a Day was intended as a funny journey through my most mortifying

SH*T HAPPENS

experiences. But we've taken dark turns as the disease, naturally, diverts us towards the more serious matters of mortality and mental health. You wouldn't pick up a book about cancer and expect cover-to-cover tumour humour. Crohn's disease and ulcerative colitis are no different; they destroy and end many lives.

In 2020 news alone, a boy died because he was too embarrassed to raise concerns about his symptoms. A young sportsman passed away from surgical complications. Another young man chose death over life with a stoma bag. And just a few months before this (in 2019), a ten-year-old committed suicide after being bullied for his stoma bag.

To anyone reading this, I hope this book has made it easier for you to chat shit, rather than go on feeling it.

Now, if you'll excuse me, I'm off to find out what shit happens next…

Open Letter: Mental Health & Misinformation

To beat misinformation, medical experts need the resources to take mental health seriously

People don't often turn to holistic, alternative medicine as a first port of call. Normally, these options are explored out of desperation. Once a patient stops feeling their voice heard, both they and their money become prime targets of those pushing untested, homeopathic remedies.

Time and time again, in scientific studies, these non-mainstream options are proven to be no more effective than placebos.* In short, the whole industry is trash. It exists to profit from our vulnerabilities and undermines the terrific work of real scientists and doctors.

Now, with NHS waiting lists reaching into the millions, urgent action needs to be taken to improve public trust in medical experts.

One problem lies in the current disparity between caring for patients' physical and mental health. My

---

* Science and Technology Committee – Fourth Report Evidence Check 2: Homeopathy.

personal experience of a life-changing, chronic disease has taught me these are not separate entities.

A problem with both modesty and arrogance

There is a reason the alternative medicine industry continues to thrive and it clearly isn't its efficacy. (At the time of writing, at least, overpriced aloe vera gels might help a burn, but haven't been found to cure cancer, or Crohn's.)

In a sense, medical experts are too modest. They are too professional, and too moral, to give false hope. They tell you exactly what they can and can't achieve for you, and then stick to their word.

Contrarily, a homeopathic 'expert' will often promise one unregulated substance offers the solution to all your maladies. You might go away believing this and experience a mild, positive, placebo effect. This obviously has no lasting benefit. Over time (and after further pricey consultations), the initial mind trick wears off and you, as patient, are back where you started, at best. The only difference being the well-lined pockets of your alternative medicine practitioner.

Such types of treatment are often referred to as complementary medicine, which is rather ironic. The whole purpose is not to cure patients. Instead, homeopathic experts sow the seeds of scientific mistrust and misinformation, before harvesting the monetary crop for as long as feasibly possible.

Scientific commitment to matter-of-fact modesty is one issue. In interpersonal relations, arrogance is another. Doctors are, undoubtedly, heroes. However, like many superheroes, they can also carry an aura of superiority. Overworked and overstretched, GPs and even specialist consultants can too easily dismiss their patients' wider needs.

In this age of fake news, qualified medics are fighting a constant battle with holistic 'doctors' and those seeking financial gain from others' ill health. Despite peddling misinformation, these business experts – because that's what they truly are – take time to make their customers feel valued. They emphasise how they treat patients as a whole body, mind and soul.

Except, they're not really helping them. They're not really treating the ailment of the patient. The patient, after all, needs a medical expert.

Now, unlike your local reiki healer, let me be very clear: I am not a medical expert. I am a science teacher and writer. What I do have, however, is a lengthy experience with an incurable disease, ulcerative colitis (UC).

Having spent recent years in and out of hospital, I've rarely been off NHS waiting lists. With a chronic condition like mine, doctors are brutally honest and modest from diagnosis, laying out the truth with phrases such as: 'There is no cure', 'Remission is the best you can hope for', and 'Major surgery is your final option'.

I should be a prime victim for the alternative medicine industry. So far, I haven't squandered any cash on it. But I can completely understand why people do. I've felt lost. I've felt abandoned. And I've felt little more than a patient number that needs to be sorted and input into a spreadsheet.

The trick medical experts seem to be missing is this: mental health and physical health need to be considered in tandem.

Let's get more than just physical

Crohn's and colitis wreak havoc on both the mind and body. At my worst, I faced up to forty trips to the toilet a day, countless new medications each week, and lost almost 20kg in a matter of months. With so much to deal with on the physical front, the mental health impacts of my illness were brushed under the carpet.

Before my diagnosis, I'd never had suicidal thoughts, and had been both ignorant and fortunate enough to have never really understood or even experienced depression. Discovering that I had a life-long condition, that was soon to change.

On the day of my first colonoscopy and subsequent diagnosis, I was sent away with a few pamphlets and a nurse to contact if my initial medications didn't work.

SH*T HAPPENS

Getting to this point had taken months of being misheard, fobbed-off, and misdiagnosed. It had taken months of calling consultants' secretaries, trying to get help. (See how much easier it is to organise a £50 acupuncture session?)

Leaving the procedure, with leaflet and diagnosis in hand, no one had prepared me for this.

Mental health side effects

Steroids soon swelled my face to almost double its normal size. I had the sweats. Sleeping more than two hours a night was a distant dream. My memory fogged and I repeated questions and conversations week on week.

My joints became so brittle I required assistance walking to the toilet. Trying to wean off them, my energy levels plummeted. The list of impacts goes on, and on.

Aside from insomnia and all manner of grim effects, steroids also gave me the shakes. I vividly remember my lowest moments. Lying alone, in the dark, dank, mould-peeling bedroom of my rented flat, after another early-hours race to the bathroom, I observed my wrist quivering. Another miserable morning of this new normal, this semi-life.

As I wrote at the time in Sh*t Happens: finally, I understood. When you are held hostage to your health, be it mental or physical, trapped in your body,

MENTAL HEALTH & MISINFORMATION

it makes perfect, terrible sense. Those blue veins tempt. There, at the surface. They offer a way out.

The real way out

Crohn's and UC both come under the umbrella term IBD, or inflammatory bowel disease. That's not to be confused with the less severe IBS, which is irritable bowel syndrome. Up to forty-five percent of UC patients and seventy-five percent of Crohn's sufferers require surgery at some stage.

When all traditional medicinal routes failed me, I had my large intestine removed. Now, I live with a stoma bag resting on my stomach in its place.

Life with a stoma bag is well worth living. On many days, it has its difficulties. But these can be as funny as they are a nuisance.

In 2020, there was news that a man chose to die rather than have ostomy surgery. Tabloid media chose to sensationalise this tragic case. Filtering through the slush of articles claiming he didn't wish to live without sexy washboard abs, this story was clearly a matter of mental health issues as severe as his physical problems. The sad truth is that many people recovering from life-altering health circumstances are given no advice on how to protect their mental health throughout.

Despite, at times, relating to that man's suicidal mindset, my writing provides an alternative, positive story of living happily with an ostomy. And I want to encourage medical experts, through reading my work, to consider both the mental and physical health of their patients. Doing so will improve public trust in the real science and the real help we are fortunate enough to have freely available in the UK.

Yes, NHS waiting times can be appalling. But that is a logistical, political, and financial issue more than it is a medical problem.

Waiting care, *and* after care needed

While waiting to see a specialist consultant, patients require advice on how to look after their mental wellbeing. Dealing with a physical condition takes a toll on the mind. It's no surprise sufferers of chronic bodily conditions are also more likely to experience depression.[*]

Some help is out there. For example, Public Health England has launched Every Mind Matters. That's all very well, but how many people – of those who desperately need it – even know it exists?

At times during the trials and tribulations of my disease, I felt completely forgotten by the system. Not enough attention is paid to the mental health impact of being diagnosed with a disease as serious as Crohn's or colitis. Clearly, much more public awareness of the support available is needed.

---

[*] Healthline: 'Manage Depression and Chronic Illness'.

MENTAL HEALTH & MISINFORMATION

With Covid-19 exhausting an already weary NHS workforce, things are not easy. None of what I say aims to deduct from the fantastic dedication of all our health workers. The issues lie in the time, freedom, and resources provided to that expert medical workforce.

As a patient, it's starkly visible just how busy doctors and nurses are. It's hardly surprising, therefore, that once you're out of sight, you're pretty much out of mind, too, until further pressing physical problems arise.

After my diagnosis, I was left with my leaflets until I returned in dire straits. After surgery to remove my colon, I had a couple of brief checks to ensure my ostomy bags were functioning. Not once was my mental health checked on.

When I faced frightening complications in the post-operative months, my GP appeared to have little understanding of how to assist. He certainly didn't have the time to ask how I was coping with it as a person. As a young man, I hadn't heard of UC when I first joined his GP surgery, but now – if I survive one hundred years as I hope – I'll live with the body-altering consequences of the disease for the remaining three-quarters of my life.

Fortunately, I've been patient. I've spent my time in the behemoth queue, and I've recently received further surgical treatment.

But in the interim, I could have easily turned to misinformed, unregulated remedies that lure so many of our most vulnerable and chronically ill. When I started sharing my writing, my first followers weren't just friends and family. I also saw an influx of influencers claiming they could cure Crohn's and colitis with their revolutionary diet plan, or monthly-billed vitamin capsules.

My surgeon informed me that most people who have surgery for bowel disease wish they'd had it sooner. But homeopathic profiteers' seeds of doubt make this seem a dreadful solution. They tell you how unnatural surgery is. How medicines are only there to fund big pharmaceutical companies. A funny argument, in truth, when those life-saving drugs are free in the UK, but the Insta-advertised remedy always carries a hefty price tag.

Diseases and misinformation ruin lives. Doctors, science, and surgeons save them. They are well worth the wait.

Medical experts must be given the funding to treat patients' mental and physical health as intertwining factors in our overall wellbeing. Until they can compete with the alternative medicine industry on this aspect of patient experience, they will continue to fight an uphill battle.

Acknowledgements

To everyone who has read, listened to, or talked about *Sh*t Happens* – thank you. My goal is to raise awareness of invisible illnesses, and you've all helped do just that.

My family and friends have been ever present, loving, and made me laugh through what has been an incredibly shit time. To everyone who visited St Thomas'– you're the best. Special shoutouts have to go to Jake for his Deliverake takeaways, and to Lottie for looking after me when I was completely off my tits on painkillers. Also to Muz and Steph for being the most entertaining of the many ward-mates I've had in hospital.

Special thanks must go to Tom Brophy for serving as both editor of the written edition and producer of the audio version of the first series (available online), to Tracey Warr for offering both editing assistance and fulfilling the writing contracts ten-year-old me coaxed her into signing, and also to James Wheeler of Perito Limited for advising me on publishing.

I've had many moments of doubt and darkness, and sleepless, lonely nights. But the next day has always arrived, with friends and family reminding me I'm not alone.

Amid all this, meeting Tatiana has left me feeling extremely lucky. If I could go back to the 'old me', newly single and about to undergo the first surgery, writing the opening of *Sh*t Happens*, I think he'd be over the moon at where the story concludes.

Find more at
jeturleywriting.co.uk
@jeturleywriting

Coming soon from Track Press Books...

Causa by J E Turley

What if your mother was gone, and two seconds of your time would have saved her?

Tiago Oliveira is left disillusioned as adult life in outback Brazil deals its first knockout blows. His hometown, Cuiaba, is the southern gate to the Amazon jungle, but there's nothing exotic in dusty streets and derelict stadiums.

A brutal attack on Tiago's mother devastates their already discordant family. The perpetrator's subsequent acquittal, on corrupt religious grounds, spurs Tiago's hunt for purpose, forgiveness, and revenge.

Wracked with guilt, and fighting to keep an emotional meltdown at bay, Tiago's chase across the globe spans Russia, London, and the depths of the *Amazônia*.